Psilocybin Mushroom

Harvest High Quality Psychedelic
Magic Mushrooms

*(A Practical Beginners Guide to Growing and
Using Magic Mushrooms Indoors)*

Clinton Myers

Published By **Zoe Lawson**

Clinton Myers

All Rights Reserved

Psilocybin Mushroom: Harvest High Quality Psychedelic Magic Mushrooms (A Practical Beginners Guide to Growing and Using Magic Mushrooms Indoors)

ISBN   978-1-998901-12-8

No part of this guidebook shall be reproduced in any form without permission in writing from the publisher except in the case of brief quotations embodied in critical articles or reviews.

Legal & Disclaimer

The information contained in this ebook is not designed to replace or take the place of any form of medicine or professional medical advice. The information in this ebook has been provided for educational & entertainment purposes only.

The information contained in this book has been compiled from sources deemed reliable, and it is accurate to the best of the Author's knowledge; however, the Author cannot guarantee its accuracy and validity and cannot be held liable for any errors or omissions. Changes are periodically made to this book. You must consult your doctor or get professional medical advice before using any of the suggested remedies, techniques, or information in this book.

Table Of Contents

Chapter 1: A Brief History About Mushrooms

The first time mushrooms were used was probably in the ancient era of chasing and assembling. As mushrooms are not able to be created right away, they must be collected over a prolonged period of time. It is true that there are only a few varieties of mushrooms available today. This contrasts with the variety of edible species. 4600 years ago, mushrooms were considered to be powerful and extraordinary. The Egyptians accepted mushrooms as plants of interminability. Pharaohs stated that only they were allowed to eat mushrooms. Romans believed mushrooms to be the food of gods. Numerous people gather mushrooms for their use. However, many fallacies are still prevalent in the current mushroom parlance.

For millennia mushrooms have been used for healing purposes by the Japanese as well as the Chinese. Lentinus Edodes and Shiitake mushrooms were first discovered in China circa 800 years ago. Exploration of the mushroom in Japan proves its therapeutic value. Shiitake was added to AIDs medications in order to boost immune, tackle exhaustion, prompt immune response arrangement to Hepatitis A; it also energized antitumor movements. Auricular polytricha, also known as "ear organ", was first created in China about 300 to 200 B.C. This is the current state of development in several South Pacific countries. Flammulina valutipes (Enokitake) has been developed for many centuries. This little-sensitive mushroom was first created on sawdust.

Many species were developed by various societies. The first mention of mushrooms being developed in Western countries was in Paris in France, in 1650. Agaricus disporus, a quintessential shop mushroom, was first found in melon crop manure. This mushroom was originally developed in open field for a long time. Then it was moved underground into caverns. Agaricus disporus was first discovered in France by the English groundskeepers. This simple harvest required no speculation, work or space. In 1865 the United States had begun mushroom development. There are two known hereditary variants of Agaricus busporus: Crimini or Portobello.

Truffles were discovered as early as 1600 B.C. Truffles were recognized as being a result oak trees in 1903. Truffles were only available in nature until the Second World War. Underground mushrooms cannot be developed in the conventional sense because they establish a mycorrhizal, or harmonious, relationship with trees. Tuber melanosporum and Tubermagnatum are the main species that have been "developed". (Both are not British). "Developing" truffles began in 1972 at an oak estate. This required 10 years or more before the primary truffles could be harvested. Numerous attempts were made to develop oaks other than their local area, but they failed. However, some

New Zealanders tried to develop truffles, and this proved to be successful. It took just five years to collect them.

Although there have been numerous attempts to develop morels in the past, it has never been commercially viable. While there are many varieties of Morchella, the most well-known is Morchella. Ron Ower created the primary Morchella, but his yields were very low in 1980. Gary Mills of Neogene Corporation teamed up with Ron. It appeared that this was a high return strategy. But it only worked for Michigan. All attempts to apply the same technique elsewhere have failed.

Mushroom Cultivation

Mushroom growing involves six stages. Although these divisions can be subjective, they are able to help you understand what is needed to set the stage. The six stages have been divided into two phases. Phase I involves fertilizing the soil. While Phase II involves treating and packaging the soil. They are shown in the order they occur, emphasizing the key features within each stage. Fertilizer can be used to provide nutrients for mushrooms' development. Two types of material can be used to fertilize mushrooms. The most commonly used is wheat straw-slept together with horse compost. Manufactured fertilizer usually uses feed and straw. But, the term also refers to any mushroom fertiliser that does not contain horse excrement. Both fertilizers require nitrogen supplements to expand and gypsum as a molding specialist. The readiness of manure occurs in two phases, Phase I & Phase II. Phase I is where manure preparation and mushroom creation begin.

Stage I - Making Mushroom Compost
Fertilizing your soil begins with mixing and wetting all the fixings. Once they have been stacked in a rectangular heap, make sure there is plenty of space between the sides. The mass fixings are regularly filtered through a fertilizer turning machine. Water is sprinkled onto the pony excrement. The turner completely blends the nitrogen enhancements, gypsum and

mass fixings that are applied to the highest point. The mass fixings allow for the development and proliferation of microorganisms. This interaction can produce warmth, smelling or carbon dioxide, as well as warm and unpleasant odours. Constrained air circulation can be used. In this case, the fertilizer is placed on a solid surface or in passages or shelters. The constrained entrance of air via a plenum and/or spouts or nozzles in the floor allows for maximum mushroom production.

Mushroom manure results from the transformation of the crude fixations into a compound. This is done by microorganisms. These situations create a food source which is appropriate for the development of the mushrooms. Without adequate dampness, oxygen or nitrogen, the interaction can end. This is why water is added periodically and the manure heap circulated air is moved through the turner. It is not common for crude materials to be used in making mushroom manure to have a negative impact on fertilizer execution. The geology of wheat straw, its variety (winter-spring), and the usage of nitrogen manure as well as plant development controls and fungicides can all impact fertilizer profitability. To limit the possibility of unwanted and possibly harmful organisms and microbes developing in wheat straw, it should be kept undercover prior to being used to create manure.

Gypsum is used in order to control the oiliness of manure. This wonder can allow air to penetrate the heap quicker, which is important for fertilizing your soil cycle. If air is not accepted, it creates an anaerobic climate. Here harmful synthetic compounds are used which decreases the effectiveness of mushroom fertilizer in developing mushrooms. For each huge load of dry fixings and gypsum, 40 lb is added to the soil.

Today, nitrogen supplements include corn distiller's wheat, soybean seed meals, peanuts or cotton and chicken fertilizer.

These enhancements allow for the nitrogen to be increased to 1.5 percent in horse compost and 1.7% for engineered. Both of these are registered on dry weight premise. To make engineere fertilizer, you must add ammonium nitrogen or urea to the soil before it can be used. This is in order to provide microflora with a fast accessible source of nitrogen for their growth and multiplication.

The size of the manure heap should measure 5 to 6 feet in diameter, 5 to6 feet high and as long as it is necessary. To frame the heap (rick), you can use a 2-sided box. However, some turners come equipped with a "ricker", so you don't need a container. The heap should have thick sides and a free middle throughout Phase 1 fertilizing. As the straw and roughage become more flexible, compactions are possible. If the materials are not as conservative in the Phase I measurements, air can't pass through the heap. Constrained air circulation has effectively eliminated the concern of an anaerobic central point in the fertilizer.

Turning and watering should take place within two to three days, except when the heap is hot (145deg F to 170degF). Turning allows water circulate air and blend the fixings. Enhancements can be added when fertilizer is turned. However, they should be added immediately after treating soil interaction. The amount and time between turns will depend on how the fertilizer is heated up to temperatures above 145°F.

Water expansion is important because it can reduce oxygen availability by taking up pore space. If you are unsure, water serves the purpose of draining at the time the heap is framed. At the hour of the first turn, water is added for fertilizing the soil. You can apply water liberally to the manure on the last turning before Phase II fertilizing it. Water dribbles off the manure when it is firmly pressed. There is a relationship between water, temperature, nutritive worth and microbial effect.

Because it is a chain, when one factor is restricting, the entire chain stops working.

Treatment of soil takes 6 to 14 working days, depending on how the material is at the beginning and its attributes. You will notice a strong, alkali scent when treating soil. It is usually supplemented with a sweet, decaying smell. Substance changes take place when fertilizer temperatures reach 155°F. If alkali can be found, this will cause the soil to become more food-friendly. Substance changes also result in heat being delivered to the fertilizer, increasing the fertilizer's temperature. When there is an intriguing degree of organic or substance action, temperatures in the fertilizer can reach 170°F-180°F. The fertilizer should a) have a chocolate brown tone; b), have soft, malleable straws; c), have a dampness of 68-74%; and, d) smell strongly of alkali. Phase I fertilizing soil ends when it has attained the right temperature, shade, dampness, and smell.

Stage II: Composite Finishing

Phase II features two key processes.

(1) Treating the soil. You must treat your soil to remove any bugs, nematodes, creepy crawlies or irritations in fertilizer.

(2) Manure Conditioning. To remove the smelly salts from the Phase 1 soil treatment process, it is crucial to condition the manure. Phase II ends with alkali that has a fixation greater than 0.07%. This can inhibit mushroom growth.

Stage II will take place in one or more of three spots, depending upon the creation framework. The manure is mixed into a wooden sheet and placed on a plate. They are then moved into an environmentally controlled Phase II area. After that, the plate will be moved to different rooms. Each room is designed to provide the right climate for the development process. The manure is simply placed on a rack or bed frame in the room used for the yield culture. The most common framework, known as the mass framework, is one where fertilizer is placed in a safe passage with a punctured ground and controlled air circulation. This is a room specifically designated for Phase 2 soil treatment. The fertilizer must be filled uniformly inside and outside regardless of whether it's in beds, plates, or masses. Since outside air will replace the smelling salts of carbon dioxide, fertilizer thickness must be adjusted to account gas trade.

Stage II treatment of soil can be considered a controlled and temperature-reliant environmental cycle. Air is used to maintain the fertilizer at a temperature that is most conducive to microorganisms' development and repeated cycles. The accessibility of usable sugars as well as nitrogen is critical for thermopiles development. Some nitrogen can also be used to scent salts. These microorganisms make supplements and fill in for the fertilizer where the mushroom mycelium flourishes. Fertilizing soil offers the advantage of treating a greater amount of manure per 2ft, compared to more expensive production rooms. The upside to burrow fertilizing is greater consistency and better utilization of automation when combined with mass production run. The danger of unwanted microbes or vermin may increase if the manure is moved from the sanitization area to the mass create run passage. Burrow treatment might need to be done in order to disinfect the soil more effectively than in-room fertilization.

It is crucial that you remember the motivations behind the second phase when trying to choose the best arrangement and system. Unwanted alkali can be eliminated. Because it is easy to de-ammonify living things, the temperature range of 130degF to 125degF is most effective. A sanitization agreement is also used in Phase II to get rid any vermin that may be present in fertilizer.

After Phase II is over, the fertilizer temperature needs to be brought down to about 75 to 80 degF. Then, it can be brought forth and planted. The nitrogen content of fertilizer should be between 2.0-2.4 percent and the dampness in the range between 68-72%. For the best mushroom yields, Phase II will require 6-8 lb per square foot. It is vital that the temperature of both fertilizer as well as manure is uniform throughout Phase II. This is because it is very attractive to have homogenous materials.

Stage Developmental

As a mushroom matures, it produces spores. These tiny spores form on the mushroom gills. These spores act in the same manner as seeds from higher plants. To make mushroom fertilizer, growers don't use mushroom spores because they sprout in an unusual way and are not strong. Mycelium (flimsy strings-like cells) is easily proliferated vegetatively with sprouted sospores. It allows cultivators the ability to reproduce. Mycelium proliferation requires specific requirements to ensure that the mushroom mycelium is not contaminated. Generating starts with the sanitization of a combination millet, water, and chalk. Rye or wheat could be used in place of millet. Disinfected horse fertiler, shaped into blocks, was used to develop produce until around 1940. After the grain has been cleaned, it is given mycelium. The grains and mycelium will be shaken multiplely over a 14-day period. You can keep the product refrigerated for a few weeks.

After mixing the fertilizer, the produce is evenly distributed on the manure. This could take quite a while. You had to hand-mix the manure with the produce and settle it in with an instrument that resembled a rake. The bed framework is now made up of generate. An uncommon machine mixes the fertilizer with the manure, and then brings it back in with small prongs. As the fertilizer moves along a transport path or is being transported into a container, it is mixed with generate to form a cluster framework. The producing rate can be expressed as a unit (or quart) for every such square feet of bed surface. One unit for every five ft2 is desirable. The rate is communicated here and there based upon produce weight versus dried manure weight.

Supplement Generation

In the 1960s, yield gains were noticed when fertilizer was added to protein- and additional lipidrich materials in production, packaging and later. The fertilizer could see a 10 percent increase in yield if small quantities of protein supplements were included at generation. The amount of supplementation and the relating advantages that could possibly be achieved were severely limited by the unreasonable warming and incitation of contender molds to the fertilizer. These limitations were overpowered by the creation of postponed disposal supplements for mushroom culture. Miniature beads of vegetable ole inside a denatured protein cover helped to eliminate the weaknesses in the supplementation with non-treated mushroom fertilizer supplements at generating. It was possible to obtain increments of up to 60%. There are now a few business supplement options that can be used for packaging or production of mushrooms.

Micro-max can also be used to alter the mushroom substrate. Micro-max contains a mix of nine micronutrients. Explorations have shown that about 70% of the observed yield increase is due to Mn. Mn has been added to deferred drainage supplements by mushroom cultivators who have begun to grow business supplement crops.

Mixture of fertilizer and manure has been done to ensure that the fertilizer and produce are level. Temperature is maintained at 75-80 degF. Overall stickiness is kept high to avoid drying the fertilizer and produce. In these conditions, the fertilizer will produce bring forth - a stringlike organization of mycelium. The mycelium is filled in all the way from a bring forth grain. In the long-term, the mycelium from various bring forth crops intertwine making a created bed of manure an organic element. After the fertilizer is added, the produce appears as a yellowish-blue-white mass. The generate creates heat and, depending on the cultivar and temperature, can cause mycelium to die or be damaged. Temperatures below 75°F allow for more product development and an increase in the time it takes to collect and bring forth mushrooms.

Phase III and Stage IV manure

In a passage, Stage III manure (or Phase II) produces run-in material. The passage can then be taken out and packed for shipment to the producer. Phase IV fertilizer can be sprayed with Phase III fertilizer and allowed to colonize its casing layer before being shipped. Both Phase III as well as Phase IV fertilization are dependent on the natures of Phase I, Phase II and III manures. Additionally, the use of Phase III fertilizer may increase mushroom quality. This is because discontinuity in the colonized fertilizer can generally improve the starting tone and timeframe of realistic mushroom usability. Mass Phase III fertilizer, which allows for an increase of harvests from the production area(s), has been more common in recent years. While Stage II can produce a standard of about 4 harvests each years, those who use Phase III mass create run manure midpoints of approximately 7.1 yields. If Phase IV is employed, you can get an additional 10-12 harvests each year.

Mushroom Assortments

The United States has three major mushroom cultivars. Each of the three major gatherings contains different confinements. This means that a producer could have as many as eight strains within any given assortment. The majority of white and grayish half-and half cultivars will be used for prepared food sources such as soups and sauces. However, any disengages may be eaten as new mushroom. In recent years, purchasers are more inclined to buy the earthy-colored varieties. The Crimini assortment has a similar appearance to the White mushroom but is richer in flavor and is more exotic. The Portobello range is a large, open and dark-colored mushroom. It can reach 6 yards in length. Portobello provides a rich taste with a substantial area.

The time needed to colonize the compost depends on the generation rate and its temperature, the fertilizer moisture and temperature, manure addition, and the nature of the fertilizer. Normally, the entire produce run takes about 13 to 20 working days. When the fertilizer and plants are fully developed, the next stage can be started.

Casing

The casing can be described as a top-dressing that is applied to the mushroom spores in the end structure. Casing can also be made with a mixture peat greenery, ground limestone. Casing doesn't require any supplements. Instead, Casing acts like a water source and where rhizomorphs build. Rhizomorphs can seem like strings or structure, when the mycelium is interwoven. There are three types of mushrooms: primordia (originals), primordia (pins structure), and rhizomorphs. There won't be any mushrooms if there are no rhizomorphs. Casing should allow for dampness to be retained as dampness is crucial for the development of a mushroom. The main components of the casing include water for the mycelium's development and improvement, protection from drying and support for the mushrooms after watering. It is important to provide the maximum yield potential by giving as much water to packaging as possible, without filtering into the essential fertilizer.

Sphagnum is the most widely used material for the casing. Sphagnum's color can vary from earthy to dark. It may also be smaller, more disintegrated or deeply burrowed. The process peat is not completely dried before transport. Wet-dove sphagnum is shipped in an unsoaked structure. Due to the higher water-holding limits, wet-burrowed is preferred by a few growers. Peat greenery is not subject to purification. It's free of microbes, weed molds, and nematodes. This can reduce mushroom yield. Mixing one 6-ft3 compacted package with water and 40lb of limestone to create a manure surface of approximately 125ft2 will give you a parcel measuring 6ft3. It should be about 2 inches in depth.

Casing inoculums (CI)

Casing or inoculums can be described as a mix of peat, vermiculite and wheat grain that has been colonized. It is blended with packaging to decrease trimming time, increase consistency and enhance mushroom dispersion. While mycelium from CI colonizes Casing Layer, its wires interact with basic mycelium. This gives rise to more yields and allows for higher harvests each year.

Casing Supplementation

Casting was the first step in expanding supplements. It was attempted for the first time in mid-1960s. Results showed that more significant supplements could be added at casing to generating than at generating. Also, the yield increments for each supplement were relative to the amount that was added. Although 100% yield increments are possible, there are certain limitations and problems that can be encountered when supplementing at the packaging. When the fertilizer is being enhanced at the packaging, it should not contain any weed molds or nematodes. These living organisms could be scattered throughout the manure if it is divided before adding more.

Casting the yield means that the manure temperature must be kept at 75°F during the first 5 days. Overall, dampness should also be high. After the casing, fertilizer temperatures should be brought down by about 2 degrees each day until the initials of the mushrooms (pins), are formed. You should apply water intermittently to raise the humidity level. This will allow you to manage the limit that is before the mushroom pins structures. An "artistic expression" is the ability to determine when, how, and how many drops of water to be applied to casing. This allows experienced producers to quickly isolate fledglings.

Sticking

After rhizomorphs in the casing have been formed, mushroom formations result. Although they are not very large, the formations can be seen as outgrowths from a rhizomorph. A pin is made when the design's underlying quadruples in volume. Through the catch stage, pins will grow bigger and expand. Finally, a capture becomes a mushrooms. Harvestable mushrooms will appear between 18 and 21 days after being casked. Pins are formed when the carbon dioxide concentration of room is decreased to 0.08 percent, depending upon the cultivar. The carbon dioxide concentration in outside air is 0.04 per cent.

Natural air presentation is crucial. This is something you can learn from your own experience. It is best not to ventilate the area until the mycelium begins to appear outside of the casing. If pin initials begin framing, it is a good idea to stop watering. The carbon dioxide will stop growing through the casing and the mushroom formation structure below the casing if it is reduced too quickly by broadcasting too early. As these mushrooms grow, they push through the caisson and become grimy with age. Too little moisture can also lead to mushroom framing. Sticking affects both the expected yield as well as the nature of a harvest, and is a crucial step in the creation cycle.

Cropping

The trimming cycle has three to five days of rehashing. There are two days in between when mushrooms can be harvested. This cycle rehashes the same thing using a musical design. Mushroom development can go on for as long. Most mushroom ranchers harvest for 35-42 days. But, some harvest for 60 or more days.

For great results, air temperatures during cropping should range from 57 to 62°F.

This temperature range favors mushrooms development. However it is possible for microorganisms to grow in cooler temperatures. It may seem strange to mention that bacteria can harm mushrooms. Irritations can lead to all-out crop failures. The primary factor that determines how long a harvest takes is how prevalent the bugs are. These microorganisms are easily controlled using social practices as well as pesticides. However, it is often tempting to keep this living organism out of the developing rooms.

The moisture level in the developing room should be enough to keep the casing from drying out, but not high enough that the cap surfaces of making mushrooms will become sticky or tacky. Water is applied on the casing to prevent water pressure from obstructing the creation of mushrooms. Depending on the drying of the casing, the cultivar and the phase of improving pins, fastens, mushrooms, each watering might contain more or less than one gallon. Most first-time mushroom cultivators use lots of water. The outside of the casing seals are sealed. This is regarded as a problem with the casing's surface. Fixed casing helps prevent the exchange of gases vital for mushroom pin arrangement. After the first break, it is possible to gauge the amount of water that should be added. If more than 100 lb are gathered, 90 Lb of water is required (11 days). These mushrooms should be removed from the casing and supplanted with water before the second break occurs.

Controlling the temperatures of both fertilizer and atmosphere during harvest is done by the outside air. The outside air helps to remove carbon dioxide radiated in the developing mycelium. The more mycelial differentiation, the more carbon is created. As more development occurs immediately after the bat, more natural atmosphere is required for the first two breaks. The developing mushrooms, the space between the delivering surface and the fertilizer level in the room as well as the quality of the natural or synthetic air, will all affect the amount of outside-air required. Although experience is the best indicator of the volume of outside air required, there is an overall guideline: 0.3ft/ft2/hr with manure at 8 inches. Outside air should comprise 50 to 100%.

Ventilation is vital for mushroom development. Additionally, temperature and muggyness must be controlled. Air can be dampened by adding virus fog or live steam to it, or simply by wetting the walls and floors. A few ways to get rid of dampness in the developing room are: 1) Allowing more outside air to be present; 2) Presenting drier outside air; 3) Moving a similar amount of outside, and heating it to a higher heat. Hotter air will retain more dampness. This reduces relative mugginess. Temperature control is the same in a mushroom room as it is in your home. Boiling water circled around pipes on the dividers can cause warmth. Hot, constrained gas can be blown by a ventilation channel. It is a relatively simple method for artificial mushroom productions. There are a few mushroom ranches that are located within limestone caverns. These stone areas can serve as both a warming or cooling surface depending upon the season. Caverns, of any kind, are not ideal for mushroom growth. Also, abandoned coal mines present too many natural challenges to make them suitable as locations for a mushroom nursery. Even limestone caverns are not suitable for mushroom cultivation. They need extensive remodeling and improvements.

A 7- to 10-day period is typical for mushrooms. However, the length of the collection depends on the temperature, stickiness or cultivar, as well the stage in which the mushrooms were picked. Once full-grown mushrooms become available for harvest, the inhibitors that prevent mushroom improvement are eliminated. The next flush then begins to develop. If the shroud doesn't get too large, mushrooms can still be picked. North American buyers want mushrooms that are tight and not too wide (Crimini), while some people prefer open tans or Portobello. The distance the shroud extends is the most important factor in determining the growth of a mushroom. It does not matter how big the mushroom is. Matured mushrooms can be large or small, but buyers and ranchers alike tend to prefer medium-to-large mushrooms.

Picking and bundling techniques can change from one ranch or another. The temperature of newly collected mushrooms should remain at 35° to 45°F. To reduce the amount of time mushrooms can be used, it is important that mushrooms "inhale", meaning they should be kept at 35°F to 45°F.

Most often, a question is raised about the need for lighting while mushrooms grow. Mushrooms can't wait for the light to help them develop. Green plants also need light for photosynthesis. The good news is that developing rooms can be made more productive by editing or collecting rehearsals.

Supplements

Mushrooms make a good supply of various vitamins and minerals. They have more than 20% RDA of selenium, vitamin B2, riboflavin (nutrientB2), and copper. Criminis contain large amounts of thiamin, vitamin B1, zinc and nutrient B6, as well fiber, manganese (nutrient B5), and folic corrosive. The good news is that mushrooms are low in calories, sodium, fat and calories.

The Biology of Mushrooms

Mushrooms form the fruiting bodies of certain higher organisms. These growths contain enormous amounts of infinitesimal, stringlike hyphae. Their accumulations is known as mycelium. It fills up surface soils, natural flotsamsam, and jetsam.

A mushroom can be described as the sporulating/fruiting body of Basidiomycetes' division. This is an enormous and varied group of over 16,000 species collectively called club organisms. Basidiomycetes have a range of types, including those that are saprophytic and parasitic as well as mycorrhizal. Basidiomycetes have been referred to as the most mature stage of growth due their complex life structures and reproducing systems. Basidiocarps refer to the mushrooms of these parasites. These designs are made by specific mycelium. Basidiocarp lasts for a relatively short time. The majority of this time is spent living in tiny, stringy hyphae. These ramify across the development substrate of parasites.

Be that though it may, the term mushrooms is used in common usage to refer the spore-delivering ensembles of different types of organisms. Particularly, Ascomycetes, or sac parasites are a few living organisms. This includes natural, palatable truffles and morels. One part of the non-Basidiomycetes varieties that make the "mushrooms".

Mysophobia, or the fear of growth, can be seen in many different ways. One example is "toadstool," a name that's commonly used for mushrooms with a high tail and large caps. Toad means "death" in German. Some mushrooms' toxic, destructive and dangerous properties could have been the inspiration for the name toadstool. Toadstools also have the negative connotation of frogs. European classic stories refer to toadstools in European mythology as areas where harmful frogs eat toxic mushrooms in the backwoods.

Despite some being poisonous, mushrooms can have many captivating properties. Mushrooms can quickly grow, so if there is sufficient precipitation and reasonable conditions, lots of mushrooms may appear. It is possible that mushrooms might have unexpected shapes and development patterns. These fascinating characteristics, along with other interesting ones, were not easily explained by naturalists at any time. As such, mushrooms have gained a great standing in certain societies. They are typically associated with cold, wet, perilous, and fiendish settings. Many societies have been open to the idea of repatriating a few different animals like bats, snakes, and creepy crawlies. Today, such social biases can be much more rare because we have a better understanding of how mushrooms and other living things work.

Mushroom use is prohibited by law

As has cannabis before, psilocybin - the psychoactive ingredient in "magic beans" - is becoming more and more common. Although the Drug Enforcement Administration lists it as a Schedule 1 Drug and says that there is "no right at this time recognized clinical use and a high likelihood of misuse", many urban communities and states are now trying to sanction and control the compound, given its ability to provide relief for patients suffering from the condition.

Psilocybin (magic mushrooms), to be decriminalized and regulated

Oregon became the 1st state to ban citizens from using psilocybin. Measure 109, which was passed by Oregon citizens, allows only professionals to administer psilocybin if a patient has PTSD, wretchedness or any other mental wellness issues. Importantly, the enactment established a managed system for psilocybin therapy in a controlled setting. Oregon's extraordinary approach is that the state didn't just decriminalize psilocybin, it also made it available to patients in various controlled settings.

After watching what happened in Oregon, many cities and states have taken the same steps. Florida Psilocybin Mental Health Care Act (a bill to allow patients suffering from emotional well-being) has been proposed by a Florida state official. Connecticut state administrators have also documented new bills to alter the law in Connecticut on psilocybin. Multiple states are currently considering comparative enactment.

Enormous Businesses and Psilocybin.

As proof, substantial cash has begun filling new psilocybin companies and set up organizations looking to upset emotional wellbeing care. Most in the thriving company accept the legality for psilocybin. It's generally right where the clinical cannabis was six- or seven years earlier. While the sports and entertainment industry is not as strong as it used to be for hallucinogenics in some cases, there are still positive outcomes from college students and state voting that will increase the availability of psilocybin for psychological wellness treatment.

How Law Firms Aid Growth in the Psilocybin Industry

Law offices have begun to create hallucinogenic law practice rehearses as another sign of the increasing acceptance of psilocybin. Because hallucinogenics are therapeutically valuable, and because many organizations are trying sell their items to the public, these practices have been driven by the conviction that acknowledgment of hallucinogenics is easier. Due to the association between hallucinogenics and drug business, as well as expected future leaps for medication for psychological well being, it is not hard to see why law firms would need to investigate the space and build connections in order to plan for a potential lucrative new market.

As well as being skilled in Psilocybin and cannabis-related legal cases, there will be a need for lawyers who are proficient in administrative work and value-based law. These special ventures frequently require help with recording applications. Arrangements for the board, settling business matters, and much more. Working with a professional who is familiar with these ventures can make your organization much more able to look at legal and business issues.

The Wide Range Of Mushrooms

Mushrooms are classified in a few categories. There is also a lot between classes. Mushrooms can fall into many territories. Mushrooms can fall into different areas, like clam mushrooms. However, they are often grown in a laboratory but can also grow wild in nature.

1) Cultivated Muskets

Developed mushrooms can only be economically grown. Mushroom ranchers have many strategies and arrangements in place to get mushrooms to the market. While many mushroom ranchers use expensive equipment, I believe that it is possible to cultivate mushrooms in low-tech ways. Cremini, Portobello mushroom, cremini, clam mushroom, enoki, and other types can all be used to cultivate mushrooms.

2) Wild Mushrooms

Wild mushrooms can be those that are collected from nature by mushroom foragers and mushroom trackers. Some mushrooms develop only on the roots of certain types of trees. Some of the most popular wild mushrooms include truffles, morels, or chanterelle. It is possible to gather wild mushrooms, provided you either have the knowledge and the expertise of a specialist.

Numerous toxic wild mushroom species can seem indistinguishable with edible wild mushrooms, but only if you know which contrasts to look out for. A popular saying goes, "There are many mushroom trackers. But there are also valiant mushroom trackers." In any case, there is no old, valiant mushroom tracking team.

3) Medicinal Mushrooms

For their therapeutic properties, a few types of mushrooms have been used for centuries. Shiitake and Maitake are some of the most popular palatable mushroom varieties that have healing properties. Others are too tough or too woody to eat. These mushrooms can be made into teas, or used in different ways.

Experimentally, restorative parasites have been shown to provide many benefits, such as reducing cholesterol and treating disease. Reishi (Chaga), turkey tail and other mushrooms are examples of true restorative parasites.

4) Psychoactive Mushrooms

Psychoactive mushrooms are also known as "magic mushrooms." These mushrooms can produce psychotropic effects. Many mushrooms contain psilocybin, a psychoactive substance. These types are prohibited in many countries. Check the local law to see if it is.

5) Poisonous Mushrooms

There are many kinds of mushrooms that can cause harm in the wild. The most deadly species, Amanita disporigera, is similar to edible mushrooms. They can mistakenly be mistaken as button mushrooms, puffballs, and other edibles at various stages of their growth. Negative mushrooms can have serious side effects, ranging from making you sick to causing irreversible damage to the liver and kidneys.

6) Useful mushroom

Some varieties of mushrooms are not meant to be eaten but can be used in different ways. Europe has used Amanita-muscaria mushrooms, particularly in

Slovenia, for years to catch fly snares. The mushrooms are absorbed by milk, which attracts flies.

They can also be used to bioremediate or clean up the environment. They are capable of separating oil and natural toxins. The parasite is also capable of improving fertilizer. Researchers are continually looking at new and improved ways to analyze mushrooms. Keep in mind that mushrooms can be used as bio-fuels.

Arranging mushrooms based upon how they grow

The ability to arrange mushrooms in classifications such as developed, harmful, wild, etc., allows us to coordinate them more logically. They are affected by how they develop and what food they eat.

1) Saprotrophic Mushrooms

These mushrooms form from decayed matter. They secrete chemicals and acid that can break down tissue into smaller pieces that they can then retain and obtain supplements from. Saprotrophic mushrooms can also be formed from wood, decaying plants, and even dead animals. Saprotrophs play an important role in the evolution of life. They are the reason that there isn't any dead matter on ground. These mushrooms transform dead material into soil or fertilizer. Saprotrophs include the most commonly recognized mushrooms we have talked about. Counting buttons mushrooms, shiitakes.

2) Mycorrhizal Muhrooms

These mushrooms can form a mutually beneficial relationship with different plants and trees. The mycelium (basically the foundations in mushrooms) can mesh with different plants to form a network. The mushrooms can provide different types of moisture and supplements to plants that they are paired with. Furthermore, as a compromise, the mushroom offers sugars.

We are only a few moments away from understanding the huge advantage mycorrhizal bacteria have on plants. They enable plants to develop faster, more effectively, and larger. It's been estimated that 95% of plants have beneficial associations with mycorrhizal fungi. You will find chanterelles, truffles, chanterelles, and even matsutake in mycorrhizal mushrooms.

3) Parasitic Muhrooms

The parasitic mushroom is not like mycorrhizal, as they simply take and don't offer anything back. If given the opportunity, a parasitic fungus can poison and kill its host plants. Some parasitic mushroom species include Chaga or lion's hair, as well as nectar growth. Parasitic plants don't limit themselves to only trees and other plants. The caterpillar-growth (Cordyceps sinusis) pursues bugs, executes and finally outgrows them!

4) Endophytes

Researchers have yet to discover the secrets of endophytic growths. They attack plant tissue much like a parasitic fungus. But, the plant seems to stay healthy and develops an increased resistance against sickness. The plant also appears to take in more nutrients without any difficulty.

Endophytes may also be considered mycorrhizal due to the fact that they can grow without any host plants. Some endophytes make mushrooms, while some others never emerge from their host until it passes away.

Endophytes continue to be studied extensively. In general, there is still much to learn about them. However, we will likely re-classify some saprophytic or parasitic organisms as endophytes once we have determined what their characteristics are.

Chapter 2: About The Psilocybin Mushrooms

A few historians have accepted that psilocybin might have been used in the past as far as 9000 B.C. North African native societies were depicted in rock art. Psilocybin mushrooms are depicted in sculptures by different people. These sculptures were made in Central America in Aztec and Mayan ruins. Aztecs used the substance teonanacatl (which means "tissues of the divine beings"), that many recognize as psilocybin. The mushrooms were used in combination with morning greatness, peyote and other commonly occurring psychotropics to produce dreams, induce a daze and invoke communication with the divine. Some Spanish Catholic minister clerics were educated about the psychotropic effects of mushrooms when they traveled to New World in sixteenth century.

However, it remains highly doubtful that psilocybin mushroom could have a long-standing, sacred history. Some believe that none of the evidence is conclusive and that individuals are finding what they need from the antiquated compositions, figures and original copies. A few current clans of Central America's indigenous people groups, such the Mazatec Mixtec Nashua, Zapatec, and Nashua have confirmed their use.

Westerners began to consume psilocybin fungus in the middle of the 1950s. R. Gordon Wasson a mycologist was traveling through Mexico to observe mushrooms in 1955. He participated in a customs service using psilocybin. It was led a Mazatec Shaman, a native people who live in the Oaxaca District of southern Mexico. Wasson wrote a piece about his discoveries which was published by Life magazine in 1957. A manager invented the title "Looking for the Magic Mushroom", and the article is the source for the expression. Wasson didn't use it. Roger

Heim, Wasson's associate had enlisted Albert Hofmann's assistance (the "father") to extract psilocybin & psilocin form the mushrooms Heim and Wasson returned from Mexico.

Timothy Leary, the most popular advocate for psychotropic medications like LSD and Timothy Leary started to try new things at Harvard University. From that moment, psilocybin became an integral part of the flower child's development as well as its quest for otherworldliness. For a long while mushrooms were often linked with nonconformity.

People are increasingly acknowledging the existence of otherworldly entities. A few people have begun to take micro-dosing of psilocybin. It is basically the burning of small amounts. They do not experience all-out adventures. All things considered they feel a lift and an increase in creativity. They also find it less stressful and more profitable. A few studies support their discoveries.

Researchers are currently exploring different methods of examining these puzzling synths. In the 1970s, there was no restriction on psilocybin other than for clinical exploration. But this has only recently been reinstated. Compass Pathways was permitted by the Food and Drug Administration to conduct research on mushrooms as a possible treatment for sadness. Scientists will combine extreme treatment with psychoactive psilocybin for better treatment-safe despair. The scientists claim that this condition affects approximately 100 million people worldwide.

Johns Hopkins University launched its Center for Psychedelic and Consciousness Research (September 2019). Researchers are evaluating psilocybin to determine if it can be used as a treatment for everything: Lyme infections, narcotic cravings, Lyme, post-awful stress issue, nicotine dependence, and many other psycho-afflictions.

There are many experts all over the world who study the possible therapeutic uses of these mysterious synthetics. Each specialist aims to uncover how psilocybin mushrooms, their mixtures, relate with our brains. Maybe their work could open doors to insight that we have yet to grasp.

Psilocybin Muhroom Cultivation

It's currently illegal to cultivate psilocybin in many countries. However, clinical researchers are working diligently to prove the clinical efficacy of hallucinogenic substances like psilocybin. These drugs will probably become legal in the near future. This way you can learn the cycle so that you are ready for them to be legal.

You might now be asking yourself how long this process takes. This is a remarkable question. Here's how it might look:

Spore immunization is required to stop spore germination -- within seven working days

Spore germination is necessary to finish colonization of your cake. It takes approximately 1 to 2 months.

Beginning of fruiting cycle -- approx fourteen days.

All things considered the cycle takes around a month to complete from spore vaccination to fruiting.

This is exactly what you'll need:

Stage one

10 sterilized vaccination bottles with a substrate. Another alternative is to have one container for every cc you put in your needle. You can also make the vaccine containers with wide-mouth bricklayer boxes, earthy colored Rice flour, or another substrate. You'll still need to adhere to an exceptional disinfection procedure.

Latex gloves

Paper towels

Face Cover (concerningCOVID19, most likely as of right now)

Scouring liquor

A needle of mushroomspores (spore niels are also available online). There are some states, like Oregon and California, that most places won't transport. I did find one hotspot for these, however. It is important to choose hypodermic needles of the correct size.

A lighter

A container of hand sanitizer. (Lysol)

Stage 2

A splash bottle

A fruiting room -- A clear plastic tub that has a top. You will need to drill 4 or 5 1/2 inches holes on either one or both sides of your developing container so that air can circulate.

Temperature and muggeriness

Vermiculite (Some producers recommend Perlite. There is a subtle difference between the two.

3-percent hydrogen peroxide

There are four main ways you can receive a benefit in your endeavors.

Cleanliness

Mugginess

Light

Temperature

As we explore the means, you will learn more about each. These are the details:

Phase 1

You'll be making what's called "a birthing cake" in Phase 1 of your development. A birthing is when mycelium completely takes over your container and twists around the substrate. It will remain together as a cake once it is removed from the bricklayer.

Sterilize. This is the number one enemy in mushroom development. It's microscopic, aggressive organisms that are responsible for sterilizing your containers. These are the reasons you will find the below-mentioned ways to disinfect containers and the atmosphere. You want to stop microscopic organisms causing anarchy with your spores, and duplicating in the containers.

Take a small, dark room in your home and make it your prep area (or secret lab).

Take one step at a time and list every thing you can. You can cover your face and go into the room.

Make sure to spray the room with the sanitizer. Now, don't forget to put on your gloves.

Wipe the containers with scouring liquor and paper towels. You should pay special attention to where the top of the container is located.

Inoculate by using your lighter to heat the metal part of your hypodermic knife until it shines a red. Commonly, hypodermic and sterile needles come pre-cleaned.

After you have cleaned the needle, don't let it fall. You can keep it there until the needle is cold.

To evenly disperse spores, shake your needle. Place the needle in the port, and infuse 1 cc into each container.

Take out any extra containers and wash your needle.

Wait. Then, infuse your containers with the water. Keep your container at 80 to 85 degrees Fahrenheit. Although this is very energizing it's also good for your health. However, please do not forget to check your containers at least once every five days. They need the dull.

Within five days or so, a fluffy, translucent substance will form in your containers. As this is a good sign, you should bounce around and perform a cheerful, happy dance. Mycelium can be seen as the white substance. Mycelium is the vegetative section of the organism. It looks like the foundations on a plant. Also, the mushroom is very similar to the blossoms on the plants. The mycelium should develop in no less than 15 days. It may take longer. Wait seven days for your containers to become 100% colonized by mycelium. Then proceed to stage 2.

Phase 2

It is an excellent time to dispose of the birthing pans. They'll be sprouting mushrooms all month.

Mycelium cakes are ready to be born. The mycelium must also have been kept in a sealed container. You'll need to give them a pleasant spray for 12 to 24hrs before they are allowed to move into their new home.

Prepare large plastic bags with lids and some sifted tap water.

Clean your hands and gloves.

Take off the covers from your containers.

Don't waste your time with the band.

To remove the cakes, you can hit the container with your hands. It might take some banging and shaking in order to get it out of the container.

Place the cake in the baggie or holder. (Cakes are very sturdy once they have colonized mycelium. Once that happens, they won't be able to break or go stale.

Make sure to fill your baggies and compartments as full as you can with separate water, then seal them. Baggies can cause the cakes to fall, so be sure to seal them well.

You can leave your cakes in your cooler for up to 12 hours. Some producers allow the cakes to rest for 12 hours and some others let them sit for 24.

After the long, cold shower, your mycelium-cakes are now ready to go into their chamber.

Prepare the chamber

With hydrogen peroxide (and bubbling) clean the compartment. You can flush the compartment with just plain bubbling.

Your splash bottle will contain 10 portions of bubbled waters and 1 section of hydrogen Peroxide or Hydrogen 202.

You can clean your Pearlite/vermiculite with another 10 to1 mixture of bubbling water, hydrogen peroxide, and then apply a layer onto the lower end of your developing room. It is important to fog the developing chamber periodically as it helps with stickiness.

Place the bricklayer container covers on top of the vermiculite. Your h20/h202 blend should be used to spray each cake. To ensure mushrooms grow well, leave plenty of space between cakes.

You might notice tiny mushrooms grow from the ground; these are called pins. They are worth celebrating.

Take a look at each cake to verify the health of your mycelium. You should find them smelling faintly like the fresh mushrooms you bought in the supermarket. If you notice foul-smelling scents, your mycelium might have dangerous microbes.

Phase Three

The cover should be placed on the developing chamber. It should be located where there will be a lot of sunlight. You will need to ventilate the area.

Support:

You should fog your mushroom twice daily with the combination of hydrogen peroxide and water for at least the next month. Your temperature and dampness should be checked. A temperature of mid to low 70's with a humidity of 85-percent is ideal. On the off chance your mugginess level might be low, you may need sprit more frequently.

Reaping:

Take your mushrooms out of the birthing tray at the stem's base and place them in a cooler with a tight seal. A "flush" is the harvest of mushrooms. You can use the cakes again and again to create different flushes.

Yield and Storage. Dosage.

Yield

Ten containers make ten birthing cookies, which will last a lifetime for most people. You can start with fewer containers which will result in more spores. Spores can remain viable for upto one year. Dried mushrooms last far longer.

Capacity

Mushrooms will keep fresh for three to fifteen days. They should be kept in the refrigerator as with all mushrooms. From there, dry them well and place them in the compartment. Now, cool the compartment and place it in a dark spot.

Portion

There is not a standard amount for psilocybin mushrooms. Therefore, the size of your portion depends on your affectability, size, and desired impact. It also depends upon the strength and quantity of the mushrooms. A mushroom can pop up suddenly, so be patient and start slowly. Remember that the effects can take up to an entire hour to begin to show. Setting and setting are as important as what you eat. There is a way to make sure you have a pleasant experience.

Just like everything else in our daily lives, there are many methods to cultivate mushrooms. After you have successfully grown a few mushrooms, it is possible to talk about all the subtleties involved in the perfect growth development cycle with knowledgeable, enthusiastic specialists. They will almost certainly be able to offer some comments.

Figuring The Psilocybin Moshroom Strain

It is possible that you will be interested in learning more about the spores of psilocybin as well as their mushrooms during your mycological research or novice microscopy. They are beautiful, natural life forms that grow in wild places all around the world, much like the spores from which they are produced. Their spores are legal in many states. However, they are illegal in the United States to produce psilocybin. It is important to be familiar with your local laws before you begin any involvement in developing psilocybin-related mushrooms. You should not touch, consume, or even connect with any wild mushrooms, except if your are a competent master and you are following the neighborhood laws.

However, ensuring that you're not overstepping any laws when considering them, psilocybin mushrooms are a captivating subject to investigate-- interesting parasites, as we've taken to calling them! An important thing for beginners in mycology is to learn how to distinguish psilocybin from other mushrooms. Psilocybin and other mushrooms will share some similarities. However, mushrooms with brilliant earthy tones will require your attention. Their stems will have a blue mottling when they are wounded. This is because of a substance reaction, where psilocybin, oxygen, and the environment reacts to each other. Last but not least, psilocybin fungi will generally have a purple-colored cover around their gills. It may also show up on the stem as a little dull purple circle.

Things to Remember Before You Cultivate

You will find that mushroom cultivation is not difficult if you recognize the potential problems. These normal problems can often be caused by trying to grow mushrooms in a way that isn't right for them. These are the most important factors to consider when starting your mushroom cultivation venture.

1. Disinfection of mushroom-developing substrate

Tainting leads to disappointment in the development of mushrooms. Tainting can result from poor sanitation. Before you begin any work, make sure to clean all surfaces, equipment, holders, and gloves. You must disinfect all substrates.

For heat disinfection, be sure to always check the pressing element when using a constrained stove.

After each infiltration, fire treat the needle.

Equally important, the workplace is. It is vital to maintain a clean, neat, and sterile environment in order to improve your chances for success.

2. Individuals with strong mentality will win in the end

First-time mushroom gardeners are always eager to produce the final product. Mushroom farming can be a very intensive process and you shouldn't rush.

Not following or making the right arrangements will result in a greater chance of defilement.

You will also experience high failure rates if you try to stimulate each stage. Let your substrate cool completely before vaccination. Before the fruiting stage begins, ensure Mycelium colonizes your substrate completely.

3. It won't bring you a fantastic result if your compromises aren't made.

There is often a need to make compromises in order to save money. This is not a good excuse when you are developing mushrooms. Even though the cost of creation can be so low, it makes sense to make sure you have the right inputs in order to increase your chances of success. If you don't have what you need to manage the development process and attempt to develop too quickly, you will eventually be frustrated.

4. Right climate for mushroom growing

Unfavorable temperatures can quickly result in disappointments. It is crucial to make sure you check the prerequisites before you start cultivating any unusual mushrooms. There are many natural habitats for mushrooms, so each individual needs to be considered. These are the main points of view:

Temperatures in the air and on the ground

Dampness

Conditions that are mild

Natural air trade

5. Learn all about thermogenesis

Thermogenesis occurs when the mycelium begins to lose its natural matter. The mushroom substrate, like fertilizer heaps will start to produce heat. The temperature of the substrate may rise above that of the surrounding air. Your substrate may cook the Mycelium, even if you are able to keep your fruiting place at an ideal heat. This could be a sign that your mycelium is cooked and will eventually die.

Here are some other things to watch out for:

There are some mistakes that can be made when growing mushrooms. Here are some simple things that will help you increase your prosperity.

Learn how early warning signs of tainting appear. It will save both time and money. You should remove any defiled things from the territory once tainting becomes apparent.

An error that can lead to too-wet or too-dry substrates is common. It should be slightly damp, but not wet. Use a delicate press to get a few drops overabundance water.

To avoid disarray, identify your containers with dates, species, and groups.

Follow the method you used to start.

It is essential that you ventilate your work space after you have finished with the spores.

It is crucial that you practice clean methods right away when you start your mushroom growing venture. Most pollution issues can be prevented by using legal methods and top-quality equipment.

You shouldn't rush your initial development. Do not rush and do not compromise.

You should ensure that your environment is appropriate for the type and size of mushroom you intend to cultivate. To keep an eye on everything, you need to monitor temperature, air traffic, light, and muggeriness.

Mycelium develops heat. Point a few degrees below ideal temperature so that you don't cook your mycelium.

Laws Guiding Psilocybin Mushroom Cultivation

Many are trying to find safe ways of venturing out of their homes in the face of the ongoing pandemic. Central Texas is known for its willingness to explore the outdoors. For some, this can mean setting up camp in nature. It is obvious that cannabis tactics are becoming more humane in Texas, particularly in Travis Hays and Williamson. What can we say about mushrooms? Are individuals facing criminal indictments in Texas for enchantment with mushrooms? The short answer: Yes, the punishments can be severe. We'll provide further details below.

What are Magic Mushrooms and How Do They Work?

We must begin with the basics. These mushrooms can also cause dreams when ingested. Psilocin or psilocin can be used to induce a feeling of high. Psilocybin mushrooms is often called:

Magic mushrooms

Hallucinogenic mushrooms

Or simply "shrooms"

Psilocybin Mushrooms in Texas Law

The Texas Penal Code, the Texas law book, makes it illegal to possess and disperse, carry, use, or create Psilocybin Mushrooms. The Texas Controlled Substance Act designates mushrooms as a controlled substances in the "Punishment Group 2A", just like other genuine drugs such as MDMA and euphoria.

Penalties or Medication Costs

Texas law considers any amount of marijuana to be a crime. No matter how little you might have carried with you a few mushrooms in your climbing backpack, you could be charged with a crime. The specific charges for possessing or attempting to possess psilocybin mushrooms (or any other type of psilocybin-related crime) vary depending on how much medication is found in an individual's property.

Texas may impose penalties for lawful offenses level medication errors.

Prison or jail time

It costs a lot to pay fines

Loss in the option of owning a gun

Obligatory medication counseling

This is only the tip.

Even though Texas Penal Code allows for violations to be punished, examiners do not recommend punishments beyond that range. Always remember, however, that the country investigators usually recommend harsher discipline in every case. If you've been charged with medication violations outside of Austin it is necessary to immediately contact a quality lawyer that has experience working in provincial networks.

Travis County Exception

Jose Garza, the District Attorney of Travis County, has been sworn-in as of January 1, 2021. Garza has pledged to decrease the number of Austin arrests for peaceful crimes and to treat drug-related problems as medical matters, instead of criminal equity issues whenever possible. His group plans to forgo squeezing allegations against individuals who possess opiate substances, like meth and break, in quantities of one gram or less. In Travis County, if you're caught with less than 1 gram of mushrooms you won't likely be arrested for Possession of Controlled Substance. In any case, a one-gram amount of the drug is not a large enough quantity to warrant criminal prosecution for illicit mushrooms.

If You Get Captured with Shrooms...

Most importantly, it's your right to refuse to permit a police officer to inspect your home or vehicle. If they ask you for your permission, you are free to say no. The Fourth Amendment to United States Constitution gives individuals protection from unreasonable searches and seizures. While it is impossible to know what is "sensible", there are some rules that can be used to decide the right level of sensibility. For instance, if a cop has a warrant from the courts or can see illegal items on display, then it is legally sensible for them to go through you. An official can request to search your property, regardless of whether or you deny that there is a hunt. You have the opportunity to prove that your inquiry was valid and reasonable. If they agree to the pursuit of you, they don't need to show that it was sensible.

If you're arrested...

It's possible to still expect the best if you get into trouble with a medication case. It can have a tremendous impact on your case if you have a qualified criminal protection legal counsel close by. For example, no matter if you were in possession of an illegal substance, like psilocybin mushrooms, a skilled lawyer might be able show that the pursuit by the cop was illegal. If the police pursuit is unlawful, all evidence that was seized can be used in your favor. You can have a lawyer advocate for you at preliminary or help to arrange a great ask arrangement, regardless of the legality of the hunt.

Here's What You Need To Know

In some places on the planet, marijuana has been made illegal and sanctioned. Texas is not one such state. Therefore, it's important that you adhere to legal indecencies. If you do find yourself in possession of the products, know that you have rights.

Chapter 3: The Psilocybin Mushroom

Seedlings

Psilocybin contains psilocybin in around 200 different types of mushrooms. They are created from spores. It's possible to obtain them legally since psilocybin-free spores do not contain psilocybin (a banned substance in the U.S.). How do you cultivate them? It is important to observe the law.

Psilocybin won't be born in a parasite until spores develop and start to create mycelium. This is what you see in the contagious strings. Mycelium forms underground in the forest or in rotting tree stumps and becomes mushroom fruiting body. Therefore, psilocybin-spores that sprout and grow into mushrooms are illegal.

Where to get Psilocybin Spores

There are many ways to remove your Psilocybin Spores. But it's easier to simply get them on the internet. Google will bring up a number of unimportant purveyors willing to sell a needle or print. A psilocybin needle with spores is basically an oral needle with water and mushroomspores. Spore prints can be described as bits of paper that have had the spores stepped upon. It is done by covering the paper with a mushroom cap and allowing the spores fall to it. Spore prints are dry and should be kept hydrated until you're ready to use them.

Individuals may purchase psilocybinspores for the purpose of studying them under a magnifying device or making mushrooms from them. Selling or buying psilocybinspores is legal in the vast majority of the United States. Georgia and Idaho qualify for exemptions. It is not illegal to buy psilocybin, but it is prohibited in Denver, Colorado and Santa Cruz, California. Ann Arbor and Michigan were also selling and developing psilocybin.

Spores

You must ensure that you obtain the spores that you request when you search online for psilocybin. This is because these spores can be purchased online. It's like wandering through the Wild West. There are no guarantees that a merchant will be able to guarantee the needles' sterility, or that the needles you receive contain spores. To make sure that you're buying a protected item there are some things you can do. Find out if there are any places that offer spores only to mycologists. This could be for training, distinction proof, examination, or inspection. Look for mushroom discussions, such as "Shroomery", and ask. The merchant may not be willing to sell you spores if the customer says they intend to sprout them or use them other than for their own purposes. In some areas of the world, it's still illegal to grow psilocybin seeds.

* Psilocybe Cubensis

Psilocybin is available in many different forms. However, the Psilocybe Cubensis mushroom is the most common, especially for the purpose of development. One simple, rational perception might be the most powerful demonstration of the force, holiness, and miracle of hallucinogenic mushrooms. Their normal development is similar to a blessing from our planet. This hallucinogenic has no equal than the psilocybin flower. It is important that we explain that "psilocybin fungi" or "magic mushrooms," could refer to mushrooms that are hallucinogenic. It is also important to note that there are amazing steps being taken in the treatment of psilocybin.

Why cubensis

Psilocybe Cubensis grows normally in U.S. spaces, throughout Central and South America. It also fills well in Australia, Southeast Asia, and Central America. Cubensis are well-known because they can be grown at home. Cubensis can flourish even under difficult circumstances. They are strong against changing conditions while delicate strains may be hurt by a slight change in the environment. The Amazonian cubensis varieties B+ and Amazonian are most loved by fledglings.

Presumably the most famous and simple psilocybin Cubensis strain.

Psilocybin Cubensis mushrooms display a distinctive appearance. They have long, winding roots and long covers. These mushrooms are an excellent choice for cultivators because they are easy to grow. Psilocybin Cubensis possess gentle strength and a variety impacts. These could include enhanced tones and visual twists. People report feeling euphoric. They also feel profoundly in control, insightful, and orderly after taking psilocybincubensis. Psilocybin Cubensis may be life-changing. However, the mushroom provides incredible opportunities for learning and sustaining your knowledge.

Two grams of dried psilocybin would suffice for a typical psilocybin dose. Two grams should be sufficient to provide a few minor effects, but not enough to cause a panic attack. The minimum recommended dosage is at least three to five grams. It should take more to experience the full power of psilocybin. They can deliver results in as little at 20 minutes. Usually, the experience lasts for four to six hour.

Psilocybe semilanceata

P. semilanceata, also called the freedom cap, a grass-cherishing plant, is known for its widespread dispersion, and simple recognition of evidence. The ringer-formed covers are not usually more than an inch wide and they only measure 4 inches tall. The covers have a prominent number and are dark chestnut with earthy colors in shading. These changes become less noticeable when they dry. It has a sporeprint that is purplish to earthy and can help distinguish it from comparable-looking harmful garden species like Pholiotina carpeta and Conocybe arpala. P. semilanceata doesn't contain any psilocin. But they do have high levels of its prodrug, which is psilocybin. The spores are often wound pale blue.

P. semilanceata occurs in most parts of the planet. They can be found in gardens, fields, and other lush terrains in the fall or late fall. They are found throughout North America, including in Northern California, Columbia, Britain, Columbia, France, Germany and Holland.

Psilocybe, cyanescens

P. cyanescens usually referred to just as cyans, is a moderate-to-profoundly intense wood-cherishing species that the mycologist Elsie Wakefield found in 1946. They have a "wavy cap", undulating (or undulated) cap edge at development. The covers are caramel-hued upon arrival and dull yellowish earthy-earthy after drying. The fractional shroud, which is weblike in appearance, quickly disintegrates with the development of cyans. They have a blue appearance at maturity like other highly-strung species, and are rich with psilocin.

P.cyanescens likes to grow in sawdust or wood chips. They often grow in large quantities, especially when temperatures fall below 50-65oF. They develop most strongly on the West Coast of the United States. From San Francisco to southern

Alaska, this is where they thrive. They are found all over the globe, in countries like the United Kingdom, New Zealand and many areas of Central Europe.

Psilocybe azurescens

P. Azurescens, also known by the "Razzies", is a rare and very powerful psilocybin-producing mushroom. It was found only on the West Coast. You can identify them by their white stems, which are topped with caramel-hued, raised leaves that reach 1.5 inches in height. This cap is covered in pellicle, a transparent layer of skin. They have a knock-like feature in the middle. Their spores are dim and dark. Other signs you are within sight of Razzies include their delicate nature and bitter taste. The seaside locations of Washington, Oregon and northern Oregon are home to P. Azurescens. They thrive in soils with sandy soils as well as in rise grasses. They can also thrive on deciduous timber chips found on adjacent shorelines. They can bear fruit from late September through early January. P. cyanescens has the ability to withstand cold temperatures like other PNW wood-sweethearts.

Panaeolus cyanescens

Panaeolus/Copelandiacyanescens or Blue Meanies is not to been confused with Psilocybe. It is a strong and loving species that lives in subtropical, tropical regions of the planet. This species develops a little, chime shaped cap at its early stage. The cap becomes arched as it grows and can grow to 1.5 creeps by maturity. The cap starts out light and earthy-colored, becoming darker with time. The stem, which is pale yellowish, can grow up to 7-12cm in length and then will turn pale. Pan-cyans are easily identified by their ebony run if you consider these traits.

People living on each livable continent have reported seeing the species. It is particularly abundant in North America, South America and Europe. It's most commonly found in Florida, Hawaii, Mississippi and Louisiana in the United States. You may also find them growing on the soil of cows and sticky lands.

Chapter 4: Growing Psilocybin

Mushrooms In The Most Secure Way

A great way to do this is to get all the gear necessary for developing your mushrooms without leaving any exceptions. For some, this may prove to be a complicated process. As you expect your mycelium will develop within the substrate, you should also accumulate spore patterns or spore tips. Regular sterilization is recommended to keep microorganisms away from the substrate.

A mushroom grow kit is a much simpler option and far more helpful for beginners. You should have a mix of filler substrates and mycelium. This is extremely helpful as it makes it possible to have the best yields. Further simplifying the interaction is the fact that the pack should be all set to create a main flush. The bag may have oxygen ventilation, but it might just need clouding. The pack must be securely closed, and kept at an ambient temperature of 28° Celsius. Use a rain jug to fog the pack. It only takes a few drops of water every day.

Mushroom Spores, Syringe

Within seven days, you will begin to see clear signs. Once the main cover has appeared, full development should be expected. After that time, the time is right to harvest thespores. The best time to do this is right before the "covers" break. When the mushroom caps are broken, this is when the spores can be released. It is crucial to clean your hands prior to reaping your mushrooms. In order to avoid introducing unknown organisms into the climate that could affect the quality of your mushrooms, it is vital to wash your hands. Your mushrooms should be carefully removed from the base.

These packs provide a few flushes, which is a good thing. You need to add cold water to the cake to activate the mycelium. Put the cake in warm water for at least 12 hours. Then, channel it. You are ready to rehash these means to restart the cycle.

How to Choose The Right Growing Environment

To start, you should remember that mushrooms are organisms. Although they're not as complex as other life-forms such plants or animals, their DNA (or cells structure) is similar. Most mushrooms develop by retaining certain supplements from their current situation (like plants). This incorporates dust from the soil, surfaces, or air. Most mushrooms are neither innocuous nor noxious at the moment. However, there are some mushrooms that produce interesting mixtures which can be very solid and give people hallucinogenic effects.

These are known as "psilocybin mushrooms". Psilocybin is the substance that causes these hallucinogenic experiences, as you can see. This compound generally produces fantasies, elation and a wide variety of strange feelings.

The majority of Magic Mushrooms originate in tropical regions such as South and Central America. These mushrooms can be found virtually anywhere these days, even in the US, Canada, Europe. They thrive in normal tropical conditions. The best way to learn what Psilocybin mushrooms you like is to have a better idea of the available varieties. Even though each one of these "shrooms" has different needs, they may all fill in comparable conditions if provided with the right conditions. These are their requirements:

Space and Pot

Mushrooms love dampness. The main purpose of a pot or space is to ensure that it doesn't dry out for too long. The space or pot should contain enough oxygen to allow mushrooms to consume the rotten natural material. You should consider a plastic pot with openings on the top, or an area that can keep the space cool and disinfected.

Fertilizer and Soil

To cultivate magic mushrooms, you need to use only one type of soil. But, for them to develop, certain nutrients such as protein, nitrogen, sugar, starch, fats and lignin are necessary. For most species, they can do this using straw manure or excreta. Some options include corn, greenery or sand depending on the species. Woody conditions are the best for mushrooms, so sawdust is a great alternative.

Lighting and air

Mushrooms are not dependent on sunlight for their development, which is a difference to other plants. To flourish, they will need some backhanded freedom. This may mean that they should have a light touch of sunlight openness. However, it is important to not allow this openness to touch their caps. This could lead to injury. They also need air. A holder that opens on the top is useful because of this. The air aids in the treatment of soil, which mushrooms love.

Humidity and water

Mycelium creates mushrooms. As it's a bacterial settlement, you can call it. It develops from dampness and mushrooms would thrive if there was a lot of it. The water should be disinfected to ensure that the mushrooms thrive. The more likely the mushrooms will flourish, the cleaner and purer the water. Faucet water, for example, may be mixed with synthetic chemicals or other substances that might inhibit mycelium's growth. A condition that is ideal for mycelium is 90% of humidity. A propagator or sprayer can help you multiply the water. However, mushrooms tend to grow faster in humid conditions.

Temperatures and Environment

Mushrooms thrive in cool to warm climates. That means temperatures between 70 and 75 degrees Fahrenheit. Mushrooms grow more slowly at lower temperatures. Higher temperatures can hinder mycelium growth. You should keep the mycelium in a cellar. This would retain the moisture and temperature with tight restrictions.

Cleanliness

Although mushrooms are natural growths, they must be kept in clean environments. It is true that mushrooms cannot develop if their environment is polluted by synthetics and microbes. It could even destroy them. It's important to protect magic mushrooms from the elements by using gloves, a facial mask and a sterilized jacket. This should help ensure sterility.

The best way to Care for Magic Mushrooms

We've covered a lot of the mindful guidance, but we need to be more specific. Here are some additional tips.

Keep pets and people away

Pets and humans both have a lot more microorganisms than we do. Because the mycelium is responsible for developing and delivering mushrooms it is very delicate. If it gets polluted it will cease making mushrooms. This is why it is important to keep your pets and family away from it.

Keep your skin clean

You should clean up any mycelium from mushrooms before you tackle it. Use protective gloves, facemasks, and a blanket to cover your head. You may need to be careful not to let dust or solid breezes into your production room. The production floor will not be affected by contamination if you're clean. As such, mushrooms will develop more quickly.

Only Use Sterilized water

Because you have to maintain at least 80 percent of the dampness in the container or compartment, it is vital to shower them frequently. But, to do that, you need to use sanitized waters. It is highly recommended that you use an assimilation filter to get rid of all germs and bacterium from the water. Then, you can securely shower it.

Let them be!

The constant touch can make mushroom development worse. It is possible for them to stop growing if they are even slightly capped. This is why it is so important to defend animals and people. However, you should not come in contact with the mycelium or mushrooms during harvest.

Be careful not to overcrowd the rooms

This is about both using a large holder and not just putting together a few mycelium cookies. The conditions should be adequate for mushrooms development. These mushrooms will not develop well if mycelium cakes are fighting for the same assets. If they are left to dry, it is the equivalent. Keep a few stems close together (3-4 each) and dry them in an alternate spot. You risk them drying out too quickly and becoming useless. Keep the mushrooms well-rested in order to prevent undesirable outcomes.

Indoor VS. Outdoor Growing

Numerous faculties believe that it is possible to develop mushrooms outside due to the fact the backwoods (or any other environment with great moisture or wind current) provides ideal conditions for fruiting. There is no need for environmental control. It's obvious that the woodland is the location where the mushrooms we produce are from. So why not start growing them there? This was the logic that led to Cornell's expansion and mushroom exploration. The project was driven by Kenneth Mudge the teacher and currently emeritus. Mudge was inspired by Agroforestry or the mixture of trees, woodlands and horticultural production. Ken researched a few varieties for close to 15 years. The majority of his research was focused on log-developed Japanese shiitake mushrooms. They immediately proved to be financially feasible. He also discovered that there are other minor species, such as wine cap, stroparia, lion's mane, and clam that can be successfully developed outside.

The log-developed, reliable shiitake can produce consistent mushrooms. This is a crucial piece of inventory for any ranch business. It is possible to "constrained", or douse, shiitake-logs with water for between 12-24 hours. This makes them more organic. This technique can be used reliably to deliver mushrooms continuously from the first week in June to the final week of October.

Controlled Environment Growing

When we can grow species reliably in a small space, we feel free to explore the world. You should also think about maintaining the right environment for different stages of production from brooding through to fruiting. In order to avoid our best mushrooms fruiting, we should also take other steps to reduce pollution in our substrates. Outdoor plantations have this advantage: it is practically non-existent.

Quarterly Willie Crosby/Small Farms

Indoor cultivation systems are commonly referred now to as "controlled weather agribusiness," which includes aquaculture, hydroponics, nursery creation, and other frameworks. Mushrooms can be made in areas without a lot of money and foundation, which is in contrast to CEA-based frameworks that are used for greens. To ensure that the desired temperature, stickiness, light, or wind stream are maintained, you need to be aware of these factors and make adjustments. Indoor cultivation is a great option because it can be used in an assortment of abandoned and underutilized ranch foundations like stables. For production, underground cellars can be easily converted to steel trailers or distribution center spaces. This framework is open to both metropolitan ranches and ranchers with limited capital.

Simple Steps For Indoor Growing

Indoor mushrooms cultivation: Psilocybe, shiitake and other species are all good options. Are you curious about how to grow mushrooms inside your house? There are many ways to develop mushrooms inside. Sometimes, it can become overwhelming and difficult to make sense of all the material available on the Internet. We will break down the different methods for creating mushrooms with a tube, tissue, or straw. We'll only cover the basics of indoor mushroom growth. These ideas are the foundation for your success in indoor mushroom farming. We can safely say you are looking for the best method to grow mushrooms inside. The 7 steps involved in indoor mushroom production can be broken down into 7 different steps. The most important aspect is to pay attention the the species of mushrooms. The goal of indoor mushroom production is usually to produce massive amounts of edible, therapeutic, or profound mushrooms. This means that indoor borders should be crossed for fruiting. Instructions for developing mushrooms indoors include but are not limited to:

CO_2-sub 800ppm - dependent upon species

Moistness Above 80%

Lighting - moderate

Temperature - Preferably somewhere between 55 to 75 degrees

If you are only filling in a small area of your home, it doesn't matter how big these boundaries are. My best way to see if these boundaries are appropriate is to take a look at mushrooms. To alter ecological controls, pay particular attention to mushrooms and how they are producing. To prevent substrate or pins from drying out or becoming searing, you will need to create stickiness. If the mushrooms have long stems, with very few covers, it is likely that they require a lot of CO_2 or not enough light. The mushroom may be suffering from bacterial development. To create a favorable environment for growing mushrooms indoors you can place the fruiting substance in a glass canister, fish aquarium, or 18 gallons. Keep the top on an inclined height. You can then fog the canister up twice daily to get a better idea of how the mushrooms look. To increase

CO2 production and light levels, the top might be removed.

Growing mushrooms indoors with a specially prepared pack

This is likely to be the easiest method of growing mushrooms inside. All the necessary preparations and immunizations have been completed. To obtain the best fruiting, you only need to follow these bearings.

Making mushrooms indoors: Preparing the substrate and vaccination

When you are ready for the next stage of indoor mushrooms development, and you are ready to immunize the substrate, it is important to initially decide on which species and how you want them to be developed. To get you started, developing clams in tissue is a great way to go. The mycelium will easily eat the tissue. It is more difficult for different microorganisms. The mycelium will acquire the paper quickly by immunizing it with shellfish mushrooms and be ready for the natural product within three weeks.

This is an excellent example of indoor mushroom development.

Straw

For some cultivators, developing mushrooms on straw can be a significant advance. However, the substrate requires a slower process and requires a bit more arrangement. Indoor mushroom cultivation has proven to be more efficient in producing mushrooms that are edible or can be sold. This technique isn't the best to commercially produce mushrooms, but it is a good beginning stage. This technique is usually straightforward.

The substrate can be treated with either heat or lime.

You can vaccinate and package the straw in plastic containers that mushrooms naturally produce from.

For three weeks, keep the mushrooms on your desk and then take them out to grow in legal fruiting conditions.

Let the sacks sit for 3 weeks, and then gather them once again.

Simple Steps For Outdoor Growing

The prospect of creating magic mushrooms can seem daunting and overwhelming to many. However, an outdoor cultivation tool could prove to be a reliable solution. This kit is easy-to-use and will provide the best results for your mushroom outdoor cultivation. The following steps will help you create your outdoor mushroom garden.

What is an outdoors cultivation kit?

Outdoor Cultivation Kits contain premium mycelium. They can be incorporated into your substrate or filled in an outdoor climate. This kit is also able to develop your mushroom fix for a good long time, even without support. This unit is essential for effective magic mushroom cultivation. It is the dynamic combinations of this mushroom, including psilocybin & psilocin that give magic mushrooms the brain softening qualities. They share a place in the Hymenogastraceae mushrooms group. They can fill up in some areas of the United States such as Washington, California and Arizona. Dried mushrooms usually have a psilocin and psilocin average levels of 1.1%. This is an incredible solid element that comes from the Psilocybe species.

You must ensure that the area you create for your mushroom fix is free of parasites or other harmful organisms. Monitoring the quality Psilocybe Azurescens is a way to decrease this risk. It will help ensure that you pick the right mushrooms.

Psilocybe.azurescens has an approximately 30-100mm cap. This shape is characterized by an intense point that transforms into a vault shape. Shading is defined as something that looks like a caramel-colored chestnut. As it gets closer to the mushroom cap, it becomes more blurred. The stripe runs from 90 to 200mm in length, with a width between 3-6mm and 20-25mm.

Simple to Follow Steps

You can get your outdoor mushroom fix by following the simple steps below.

1-liter plastic holder, with cover

10-liter container of little-beechwood chips

1 medium-sized cardboard bag (greatest size (30H x 30Wx15D).

1 plastic packet

1 family fork

1 enormous pail

Acceptance to bubbling Water

Guidelines

Fill the 1-liter plastic holder half-full with beechwood pieces.

Fill the 1-liter plastic bag (currently filled with beech chip pieces) with boiling water. Allow it to cool for 12 hour. Let it cool. Once it is cooled, pour the excess water out.

After washing your hands thoroughly, add the mycelium holding substance to the plastic wrap. By gently pressing the mycelium, you can break it up with your hands.

Uniformly transport the mycelium in the 1-liter holder that stores the clammy hardwood chips.

You can discard the entire plastic bag using a fork that is perfect for family use.

Once all the ingredients have been thoroughly blended, cover the wood chips using a layer wet cardboard. Place the cover of a holder onto the top. Your mycelium needs to breathe. The top acts like a barrier to protect you from unknown elements.

Place the holder on a territory free of residues for two months. Make sure that the territory contains no residue and is free from light and warmth. Mycelium will turn white and wood chips are indicators of full immunization. This is safe to place outside.

Put the remaining 10-liter box of beechwoodchips into the big pail. Fill it up to 3/4. The wood will bubble when you lower the water level. Let this cool for 12hrs, then channel.

The medium-sized cardboard boxes should contain the clammy and immunized woodchips. Combine them with a spotless family knife to ensure that they are equally distributed.

To increase your chances at a fruitful flush, cover the box completely with soil. The crate should be kept out of direct sunlight.

AFTERCARE

Once the perfect territory has already been chosen, the actual fix can develop and flourish without the intervention of humans. If you want to create ideal development conditions, ensure that the land is constantly sodded. For a quick check, place your finger in the soil for about two to three cm. To cure dry dirt, you can add water. The final step is to protect your soil against ice. This interaction can be done in a straightforward manner. You can cover the developing area with a layer of wood chips before the period of ice.

Chapter 5: Indoor Lighting: A Need

Some mushroom species don't need light at all for development. Others, such as the hallucinogenic Cubensis mushroom species, require much more light to grow and develop sound fruiting body. All things considered these conclusions don't reflect the true amount of light magic mushrooms require. Continue reading to learn everything you need to know about lighting in your next mushrooms development.

How do magic mushrooms get grown?

To grow magic mushrooms there are seven stages: planning (immunization, colonization), arrangement of the development room, fruiting/re reaping, and drying. Robert McPherson in 1991 created the PF Tek method for home-developing.

To create mushroom fruiting bodies, you must start with mycelium. To avoid tainting, producers will fill the containers with a combination substrate. After infusing mushroom spores into the substrate, they allow it to rest in coordinated daylight for 7-14days while mycelium grows. The perfect time for the sticking period to begin is after the container has been colonized fully by mycelium. Pins are viable clusters of mycelium which eventually turn into fruiting body. Containers must be kept at a comfortable temperature, and should be exposed to the sun for this interaction. Sticking takes around 5-30 business days.

After adhering, the mycelium eggs can be moved into a simple holder (similar to a terrarium). You can cover the holder in 1.5cm layers of perlite or dirt pellets and then move the mycelium-cakes inside. Within the next 7-14 day, mushrooms fruiting bodies should appear.

* How To Choose The Best Grow Light

What type of lighting best suits magic mushrooms?

There are many opinions as to which lighting type is best for magic mushrooms. While some producers prefer the use of explicit LED lights, other growers rely on regular sunlight. Although mycelium is not dependent on light for development, artificial or natural lighting is essential to complete the cycle and guide the growth.

Some growers prefer fluorescent (CFL), lighting to cultivate their mushrooms. Artificial lighting can provide mycelium with the necessary light even without any natural daylight.

While choosing a developed light source for shrooms, it is important to consider heat and light. Magic mushrooms will prefer a light that registers close to the blue finish of a range. This is similar in style to fluorescent cylinders that emit light in between 6,000 and 7,000 Kelvin. Radiant lights are also not recommended as radiant light can emit a "red" glow in the low range of about 3,000-3500K.

Most sound mushroom producers say they can grow sound mushrooms with only natural or indirect light. Mycelium can grow in a very small amount of light. You can place your terrarium/developer pack anywhere it gets enough sunlight or room lighting. Many mushroom producers agree that the best light source is the sunlight that comes through a glass window.

How much light do your mushrooms need?

There are contrasting opinions among cultivators about this issue. While some producers prefer 12/12 lighting, others prefer to give their mushrooms less light. A 12/12 timetable will ensure mushrooms get the right amount of light. To be fair, excessive light would not be beneficial and fruiting interaction could be achieved with much less lighting. The danger of exposing your mushrooms 12 hours a day to light may be present. An extended exposure time is permissible for lights less than 7,000 Kelvin. If your light is too intense or may damage your substrate you can secure limit it to 3-4 hours per days.

Distance of lights from a substrat

Too many lights near your terrarium/mycelium can lead to excessive heat, and possibly even death. Particularly if you're using highly developed lights, be sure to leave plenty of space and to monitor for light damage.

Maximizing the Potential of Your Environment to Grow

If you've ever worked on food creations, you'll know that satisfying a task correctly expands the flavor. You can now trade in the flavor for a independent hallucinogenic trip into your psyche. A mushroom gather can produce lasting changes. It's more difficult than creating soil products to develop organisms. The latter can thrive in unsanitary, microorganism rich soil, and will adapt to climate changes, temperature fluctuations, and other environmental conditions. Interestingly, mushrooms need to be given clear boundaries before they can develop. Parasites may be created within the body by imitating the exact conditions they are required to live in. By creating them in high levels of muggeriness that are difficult to defile, this is possible. PFTek can be used for creating a perfect, humid climate. A developed pack makes things much simpler.

What makes parasites different from the plant realm are their life cycles and methods of propagation. Before you start growing mushrooms at your home, it is helpful to get a basic understanding of this interaction. The DNA that makes mushrooms is known as spores. These are tiny bits of DNA. Spores look a lot like the seeds that are produced by plants. When the conditions are right, they release small strands tissue called hyphae. This cycle may lead to germination of plants. Every hypha carries a single core. The point at which two viable, viable hyphae are merged from different spores is when they mate. The cores from both parents will be preserved by the merging of hyphae. This creates a creature capable of reproducing itself. Mycelium is made of more hyphae. This web-like structure disperses compounds into climate and remotely processes nutrients. Mycelium has a very sensitive response to outside influences. Primordia develops when mycelium has run out of food or is exposed too much light. Primordia are youthful mushroom fruiting organisms. The most ground pins mature into fully-fledged, leafy foods capable of delivering spores. The cycle is re-started from the beginning.

Proper Psilocybin Mushroom Maintenance Your elbows are not only helpful for others, but you also have the benefit of wheezing. You can be sure that your little companions will be grateful for any distance you take from the shroom. Put it all together and do the same while exhaling. It is likely that it won't matter considering that when we inhale out, tons of small particles are released into the oxygen in our nostrils. One-third of these fine particles are spores. This is the'seeds' of different growing species. Shrooms can be very sensitive to rivalry among different growths when they are developing their unit. If the spores arrive on the pack and are able to feel at ease on the warm, soggy bread, it's possible for them to grow quicker than the shrooms.

There are three colors: green, dark and dim.

Is there any dark, green or dark elements on your substrate? It is bad that the pack isn't completely grown. Are you seeing a white cushion with blue-green wounding around the shrooms? This is amazing! This proves that psilocybin has a market. It's very blue in color. What are you going to do with the unit? You might find another organism more at ease in the newly developed unit than shrooms. Imagine a jungle gym set up for children. It would include climbing equipment and a group primate friends. There are very few children who might need to play in this jungle gym. We need to make sure the parasites of the parasite realm don't have access to the famous climbing outline. Would you like to share your knowledge? Peruse on!

It is important to work cleanly

You can work with mushrooms in an open-heart setting. Use care, precision and soundness to ensure a germ-free environment. This will lessen the likelihood of green, black, or dark growths profiting by a nibble on the supplemented material. For instance, continue as follows: Use clean gloves to protect your hands when you're moving air through the unit, or gathering shrooms.

Focus is key when working. Make sure to clean your hands well with hand alcohol.

Use a fork to poke holes into the cake. Pour some bubbling water in a bowl. Put on sterile, disposable gloves

Make sure to clean the shroom unit's exterior and cover thoroughly. You can wash the top with hot water. Hot or bubbling water should not be poured into the assembled unit. This would be dangerous for the shrooms.

You can also clean water used for saturating the developed pack by bubbling it first, and then allowing the water to chill (important!).).

Shroom developed pack - Increasing the yield

You most likely have had enough counsel on how to work purely. You are now ready to ask: How can you create more shrooms. There aren't any best-in–class strategies for weed growth that you could try at home. The best answer is to make the conditions as ideal and pleasant as possible. So what are the best conditions for shrooms to thrive in a complete shroom-developed pack of shrooms?

Temperature: Shrooms prefer temperatures of 23.5deg C. The normal room temperature is between 19-21 degrees. This isn't too high for shrooms. They should be ready to go when the temperature exceeds 20 degrees. But, they may take longer and will likely be more modest than you think. It is safe to use an infrared warming blanket that has been precisely modified. This makes shrooms develop at room temperature. The tangle won't make your cake feel warm or too hot but it will heat up the warm radiation to bring it up to the correct temperature. The higher the temperature, both the mycelium (and shrooms) develop more slowly. If you are not developing it, this is why you need to keep a pack in the cooler.

Stickiness-- It's unlikely you realized that organisms are attracted to moist spots. Shrooms do well with relative stickiness at around 90%. It doesn't take much science to do this. Each pack contains a plastic bag that can be used to store your shroom units. You fill the pack with water. The water gradually dissipates. The infrared warm tangle also helps. The dampness will increase if you seal the bag with the paper pieces that are also included. It's easy. The following point is more of a challenge.

Fresh air is essential for mushrooms. Natural air is a necessity. To achieve the ideal balance between dampness and air outside, open the pack each day. Be aware that the pack can be inhaled.

You should not expose your unit to sunlight/light. Temperature changes are too much for mushrooms. The plastic bag that they are in looks almost like a nursery during daytime, especially because it is placed near the window. They can shrink quickly when they are overheated, and then develop into huge mushrooms. Your magic mushrooms should be placed in a well-lit area once the primary little mushrooms (pins), have appeared. This typically takes about 15 days. Tip - Magic mushrooms do well under blue light to enhance their yield. It is possible to explore many avenues for it if you have cool-colored light.

Add a bit of water to keep the mugginess at its best in the provided sack. This is a good time to reap your fruits. The cap should not be allowed to break.

It is not good to have huge mushrooms. But, having more mushrooms is a positive thing. Don't let shrooms grow just for the sake of gaining more weight. Shrooms can lose strength when the cap expands. Shrooms should always be harvested with an eye towards strength and not on who is thickest or longest.

Chapter 6: The Advanced Methods

Of Planting Psilocybin Moshroom

Indoors

Although psychedelics are often criticized from the mid-1970s for a variety of reasons, most commonly because they relate to legislative issues. Recently, however, the perspective surrounding psilocybin and magic mushrooms has become more flexible. People are becoming more interested in how to create magic mushrooms at home. Home development can provide a consistent, reliable supply of mushrooms without the dangers associated with picking from the wild or buying them from unknown sources. As well as being a challenge, it can also be fun to figure out how to grow your mushrooms. This could lead to a career path for many who choose this route.

Two methods are available to help you grow psilocybin psilocybin. One is to use a

Psilocybin Growkit and the other is to start from scratch with the PFTek Method. The PFTek Strategy is an outstanding indoor mushroom growing method. It's simple, just like any other thing. You can get decent results with this technique. And it can make your life very simple. The best thing is that it uses products that are readily available at any supermarket or agriculture store.

It is not easy to grow mushrooms. There may be some setbacks along the way. For successful first development we will walk you through everything. You may not be able to grow full-scale crops without any preparation. A sterile, higher-reach kit is an option.

Growing your own cannabis using a grow set

If you are a beginner it might seem scary to start an activity that is fully developed without any preparation and no knowledge. It can be challenging to develop mushrooms. I'm glad we were able address some of the issues. Before you start developing your first batch of mushrooms, it's a good idea use a well-developed pack. This will give a good idea of how mushrooms are made, what they look and don't like, as well as give you an understanding of the basics. Although these units are relatively easy to use, there are some issues with pollution if they aren't used properly.

Starting from scratch

This is the first part of the PFTek process. The PFTek method is an excellent indoor mushroom-development technique. As with any other thing, once the strategy is understood, it's very easy to get decent covers. Even though it may seem small, it can be quite rewarding. The best thing about this strategy is that it can be used with things you can find in any grocery store or cultivation center. We'll cover everything you need to start.

You'll need supplies

It is essential that you have a few basic items in order to start your own home mushroom production business. The majority of them can be found online. All the other products can be found in your local retailer or on eBay. After you have purchased all the basics supplies, you're ready to move onto the next stage.

Tip. The supplies below are sufficient for 1 container. If you are looking to build larger or smaller containers, you can change the fixings.

Hardware:
Mason Jars with Lids for 4 Wide Mouths, each 16 ounces
Measuring Cup
Sled and Small Nail
Mixing Bowl & Spoon
Sifter
Perlite
Rock-solid Foil
Cooker's pressing factor
Micropore Tape
50 -100L Plastic Storage Box
Hower Bottle
Glove box (discretionary though strongly recommended)

Fixings:

Spore Syringe 12cc

Organic Brown Rice Flour - 60ml

120ml Medium & Fine Vermiculite

Refined Water or Filtered Water

Gypsum and Instant Coffee

Sterilization:

70% Isopropyl Alcohol

Lighter or Propane Torch

Air Sanitizer

Latex Gloves or a Mask for the Face

* Using The Greenhouse Method

What are the requirements for mushroom development in a Greenhouse The best ways to grow mushrooms in a Nursery are by establishing the right conditions for fruiting. Without the proper temperature, humidity, wind current and wind, your mushrooms will become dry and unproductive. It is important to provide enough air and keep the mugginess of your mushrooms high. Different mushrooms have special ecological requirements. If there is enough space available, you can adapt it to the specific species of mushroom you are trying to produce. Some mushrooms are not able to grow well in darkness. This will require you to make some changes in your nursery to reduce the amount of light that is available.

The best gear and instruments

You can improve your mushroom game by purchasing the above.

4-level nursery

This will make it possible to regulate the climate of your mushrooms. It takes up little space and can also be used outside or inside your nursery. It can be used to accommodate many plates and squares. The nursery can also be equipped with a humidifier. This can be automatized to save you time and effort, as well as avoiding splashing too often. This 4-level nursery is available online.

Humidifiers

You can use a humidifier to regulate the nursery's mugginess. You can use a humidifier or fan in your nursery. If the humidifier doesn't have one, make sure you open it a few times a day to let in some natural air. The humidifier fan introduces fresh and wet air to your chamber. Ultrasonic humidifiers produce an easily visible stream of fume. Cool fog humidifiers are simple to use and produce a steady stream of water. To prevent contaminants getting in, ensure that you clean your humidifier often.

Hygrometer

A hygrometer can also be used in mushroom cultivation. Humidifiers are able to make a lot dampness. More often than you might think, humidity needs to be kept at around 80%. The hygrometer will allow you to check the humidity level and adjust your humidifier accordingly.

Channel fix sacks

To properly sterilize the mushroom development process, you must first wash it thoroughly. Channel fix packs prevent contaminants from reaching the substrate. Without channel patches it is difficult to control a high production medium and get high yields from exotic mushrooms. These packs disinfect and perform barometrical heating to ensure that the product is sterile.

Liner

A liner for mushroom gardens is necessary to ensure total cleaning. Barometrical is the most effective and moderate form of steaming. It effectively cleans and prepares the substrate for the desired mycelium. You can also use it to clean items like containers.

Developed light

A variety of lights can create the perfect lighting conditions for mushrooms. You just need to be careful not to give it too much heat. A thermometer is a tool that allows you to identify the temperature in your soil and chamber.

Warm tangles

Warm tangles may be bought and used. It keeps your body at a comfortable temperature. These cushions are also easily reusable and cost-effective. These cushions will help you improve your harvest, in summer and in winter.

The variety of mushrooms you can grow in a Greenhouse

While it might be difficult to select the right species, especially if you are just starting, Shellfish and Culinary mushrooms may be worth your time. Shellfish mushrooms can be grown in a greenhouse and are without a doubt the easiest species. Its name comes from the way it looks, not because it has a taste like a shellfish. It has a similar appearance to clams. In one day you will be able to master all of the important information regarding developing clams mushrooms. They are fast and practically indestructible against competing creatures. They can create many different substrate bodies.

Vaccination

Incorporate the generate with the substrate material. It's usually straw or fine wood particles. For great wind current you can even put it in packs with small openings and place them on a rack in the nursery.

Brooding

In a dimly lit area, keep the temperature between 68F and 75F. This is the beginning of the main development phase. The product takes only 14 days to grow a complete snare full of root-like mycelium string.

Fruiting

The colonized vegetables will be the first sign that your mushrooms are ready to start producing fruit. It must have oxygen, low levels of light, high dampness, normal temperature, and low-level sunlight. At this point, it will show the mycelium. This stage is crucial for mushroom development. Once the pins appear, this is the best second stage. Water and enhancements from your mycelium should be given to the pins. These tiny pins can quickly grow into full-size mushrooms in just 5 to 7 day.

Chapter 7: Using Hydroponics For Psilocybin Mushrooms

Mushrooms have chitin in them rather than cellulose. They are composed of the same structure as most herbaceous herbs: chitin. Chitins are string-like strings called hyphae. They have a long shape. They look very much like parts of a tree or a collection of roots. A mycelium is an arrangement of hyphae. Mycelium is the actual body of an organism. The mycelium's sexual organ, or fruiting, body is represented by the mushroom we see in the ground. It transmits the necessary spores for multiplication via its gills under its mushroom cap. Making mushrooms requires two separate hyphae, which means the home producer must immunize many mycelia to a developing medium.

As with normal aquaculture mushrooms spores require a growing substrate. Once the developing medium has been immunized against spores the mycelium will form, meld, colonize and colonize it. In order for this to happen, the developing medium must have supplements. This is because mushrooms do not make their food unlike plants.

Setting Up Hydroponics System For Psilocybin Mushrooms

Vermiculite can be used as a medium to grow mushrooms in hydroponics. Vermiculite is used to make a variety of supplements. It's mixed with rice flour of earthy color and a small amount water. Finally, it is made into a dish.

A mushroom hydroponics farming framework consists for most of;

A little tank full of extended dirt total rock

Water radiator

Moisture check

Vacuum device that can be used with an Air Stone.

The water radiator and the air stone are located at the tank's bottom. These stones are then covered with stones. Finally, the water is completely submerged in water and the vaccinated vermiculite cake is placed on top. The air channel will allow air to be taken through the rock and used to heat the water. If the tank is kept at 70% stickiness for six hours each day, the oxygenated environment of the tank will enable the mycelium in the tank to turn on for fruit and mushroom growth.

This technique is much more efficient than conventional hydroponic mushroom farm. The best part about developing it yourself is that you don't need to use pesticides.

Hydroponics - Nutrients

Supplements that are given to organisms will be used up as their sole source for energy. The organism life support system is similarly supported. This means that mushrooms should be given sugar or carbs to help them thrive.

How to Care Your Hydroponics - Grown Psilocybin Muskhrooms

"Birth," the colonized substrates. Open each container and remove the dry layer of vermiculite. Turn each container upside-down and tap down on a clean surface to deliver the cakes.

Make sure to dunk your cakes. Wash each one separately with a virus tap. Place the cakes in a container or other area and fill it with lukewarm. They should be just below the surface if you have another pot or comparable hefty material. Allow the cakes and other ingredients to rehydrate for 24 hours at room temperatures.

Roll the cakes. Once the cakes have been removed from the water, place them on a clean surface. Fill your perforated bowl completely with dry vermiculite. Your cakes should be rolled separately to cover them with vermiculite. This will prevent the cake from drying out.

Transfer to the prepared chamber. Place them in the chamber. Place the cakes on top. Turn the cover to close.

Optimize and screen conditions The cover-up can be used up to six time per day, particularly after moistening.

NOTE: FLUorescent lighting is sometimes used in a 12-hour cycle by some producers, but it's fine to have erratic lighting during the day. Mycelium just needs very little light for finding the outside and where to bring forte mushrooms.

Outdoor Psilocybin Muhrooms: Where to Find Them

Even if your kit is fully developed, it's very easy to make magic mushrooms. You should be aware that spores are not the easiest way to grow mushrooms. If this is the case, it may take more work. You must ensure that your mushrooms are free from any pollution. This is why it is important to find a safe place where you can grow mushrooms without exposing them to dangers. It's not necessary to stress about the development of your mushroom plants by setting up an open-air area in your nursery, terrace or garden. Instead, expect excellent yields.

There are many options available if you do not need a nursery to produce magic mushrooms. You could find an isolated spot in the woodland. This gives you the benefit of mushroom spores being freely distributed around, creating an "icing spot" where mushrooms can develop normally over the long term.

Circuitous daylight

Magic mushrooms love places with continuous daylight. Although they enjoy the sun, their eyes don't care if it is blocked. It's ideal to locate a place where your mushrooms can still get enough light for the day. In nature, mushrooms often grow in dense areas where grasses meet bushes. To locate a particular spot, you can search for these types of territory.

Swales and Slants

Common slants as well as swales are where mushrooms fill in naturally. These spots have often a subsurface flow of water which greatly helps the development and growth of the mycelium.

* Psilocybin Mushrooms: Private Gardening Method

Are you wondering how to grow magic mushrooms for your back yard? These are the basic and more advanced steps that will make your garden grow magic mushrooms. Psilocybin/Magic mushrooms can be easily developed if you're able to manage the stickiness and dampness of the environment by creating great conditions. They can't wait for daylight to develop. It all starts with a spore, which develops into one mushroom. A few mushrooms are then created later. Let's have a look.

Growing Magic Mushrooms: Prerequisites

For development and food, mushrooms don't need as much light as other plants. This is why a cellar, or any other dim area, is the best place for them to be developed. They need moisture because it holds their spores' dampness.

Dampness. Like all parasites they can thrive in clammy environments. For mushrooms to thrive, they need moist developing media like fertilizer and compost. Likewise, fog forms dampness.

Temperature is important for magic mushrooms development. It should be between 65-75F (18-24C). You should keep them out of the cool wind, dry air and heat as it can cause their death or hinder their growth.

Supplementation: Mushrooms require starch, sugar and fats to grow well. Use fertilizer that is made from straw or excrement to provide these essential nutrients. These materials may not be available to you so you can use sand, peat greenery or corn. They can also be used to remove basic supplements from logs.

Choose a Growing Spot Consider these Factors

Choose an area where the air temperature is between 55 and 70 degrees Fahrenheit. The stickiness should be between 80 percent to 95 per cent.

Woodboard mushroom beds about 50 inches across and 6-8 inches down should be assembled.

Pick the length that fits most into space.

To prevent seepage and ventilation, leave 1-inch holes in lower parts of the planting containers.

Use fertilizer made up of pony compost or roughage, poultry fertilizer and ammonium citrate.

All fixings should be placed in the planting pots. Once the soil is moistened, you can use water to make it a damp wipe. Allow the mixture of ingredients to go into compost for 14-days, turning it once a day and wetting it frequently.

Watering

Magic mushrooms grow well indoors, especially when they are in controlled conditions. They require a consistent soggy climate in order to thrive. That means they need water daily. The amount of water you use is as important as the method you use; too much water can kill the mushrooms.

Wet Substrate

Before you plant mushrooms your soil must be moist. To grow, mushrooms require a high-quality fertilizer. Horse excrement with straw is an excellent substrate. You should soak the heap in water until it is completely saturated. Then, mix the water throughout. After a few days, you can turn the heap by adding water. This will ensure the heap stays slightly clammy. After a while you will notice a slight sweetness in the manure. Make sure to add more water right before you place the manure inside the box. You want the fertilizer to be in a form that can be easily pressed with two to three drops water after you have gathered a small amount.

Spawning is on the horizon

Once you have removed the insane manure, mix it with the main 2-3 inches. The fertilizer must be clammy to encourage contagious strings (mycelium) to grow. Use a few layers paper to press the manure onto a flat surface. It takes half a months for mycelium to grow. So, use a shower bottle to spray the paper for two to three days. Avoid putting water on the manure and paper. You can create wet spots in the fertilizer which won't support mycelium growth.

Packaging Coverage

If the paper shows white parasitic webbing, add packaging to encourage the mushroom to come out. Add equal amounts of peat or nursery soil to the paper. When you press it, add some water until you see a small number of clusters. After you have placed about 1 inch of packaging on the mycelium and fertilizer layer, wet the packaging again with more water. The packaging should be kept clammy, but not too wet. The development of mushrooms takes approximately three to five week.

Humidity

Stickiness is the level of water visible throughout the mushroom. To thrive, you need to have high levels. It is recommended that mushrooms be grown at 65 to 70 degrees Fahrenheit.

Germination Period

At this point you may be wondering about the germination cycle. This is an astonishing question. Here's how it might turn out:

Spore immunization against sporegermination -- within seven calendar days.

From spot germination up to complete colonization of a cake -- approximately 2 weeks to about one month

Beginning of fruiting cycle -- approx fourteen days.

Everything being equal, it takes around a month to produce fruit from spore vaccination.

Guide For Harvesting

1) Watch out to look for natural product: Your mushrooms or natural items will initially appear as tiny white knocks. They then turn into "pins". They will be ready for harvesting after 5-12 working days.

2) Choose your natural foods: When the cake is done, cut the mushrooms around the cake. It's important to not wait for the mushrooms to mature as they will eventually lose their strength.

Don't forget: It is best to gather mushrooms before the shroud begins to break. These mushrooms will have light, tapered mold covers and covered grills.

Preservation and Storage

Psilocybin will go sour in half a week in a refrigerator. Preserving them is an option if you want to use them in micro-dosing. Drying is the best way to store them for long periods. If they are kept in an area that is cool, dry, and dark, this will help them last for years. Lo-fi is a way to dry mushrooms. You simply need to leave them on a piece parchment for a few more days. However, they won't get "wafer dried" by this method. The problem is that they won't break if you twist or twist them. Therefore, they will remain damp. You may notice a decrease in their power depending upon how long you forget them. The most effective method is to use a dehydrator, although this can be costly. The following is a good option:

Your mushrooms should be air dried for 48 hours in perfect conditions with a fan.

You can place a layer o desiccant onto the foundation of an impenetrable holders. The most readily accessible desiccants are silicagel cat litter and anhydrous sodium chloride. You can get these products at local tool shops. Use a wire rack, or a similar set-up, to prevent mushrooms from coming into contact.

You will need to mastermind the arrangement of your mushrooms on the rack.

You can wait for a while, then you can test to determine if they are wafer dry.

Move the sacks to their maximum capacity (e.g. Ziploc) and put them in the cooler.

What Does Psilocybin Do?

Psilocybin is a stimulant medication that can make it seem like you have real visions and hearings. The ecological factors that cause the effects of magic mushrooms in any given case are generally considered to be exceptional. It is well-known that mushrooms are associated with deep encounters, self-disclosure, and profound encounters. Many agree that magic mushrooms and mescaline can help people reach their highest potential. Some use magic mushrooms to feel rapture or association.

The body's psilocin converts to the psilocin in mushrooms. This has been accepted as a mechanism for altering and strange feelings. The effects last anywhere from 20 to 40 mins to start, and can last as long as 6 hours (which is roughly the time for psilocin processing and excretion). The impacts of magic mushrooms are caused by several factors: quantity, weight, character and climate.

Experts Speak

The demand for Psilocybin mushrooms can be quite high. They are known to incite uneasiness. Informally, "terrible excursionson" is what most medical clinic affirmations are connected with when magic mushrooms were used.

Recently Approved Applications

Magic mushrooms have long been used by Native Americans of America and Europe for their spiritual and restorative properties. John Hopkins University scientists recommended that the medication was renamed from Schedule I into Schedule IV in 2018. This was to allow for clinical use. Studies have shown that Psilocybin can treat mental issues such as anxiety, depression, tension, and nicotine compulsion. Denver became the first place to allow the use of mushrooms. Oakland joined in a little over a year later. However, this doesn't necessarily mean mushrooms can be legally used.

Common Side Effects

All psychedelics are prone to causing emotional and mental issues. Young people are more likley to take magic mushrooms when they're consuming alcohol or any other substance that is related. This increases their vulnerability to mental and other health issues. The amount of psilocin, psilocin, and magic mushrooms are not known. In fact, mushrooms exhibit a dramatic shift in the levels of this psychoactive substance. This makes it extremely difficult for users to identify the intensity and type of "trips" they may have.

Magic mushrooms can induce a gentle excursion that makes the user feel lazy or loose to an alarming degree. This could be accompanied either by mental trips, dreams or frenzy feeling. Convulsions may be possible from magic mushrooms. Magic mushrooms can have both mental and physical side effects.

Signs that you are using

Laziness

Migraines

A larger pulse, increased circulation strain, or higher temperature

Coordination is lacking

Muscle shortage

Frequent Sickness

Yawning

Mental impact

A bizarre feeling of time and spot, as well as reality

Elation

Visual impairment (visual or audible)

It is possible to experience contemplative (otherworldly), encounters

Frenzy responses

Psychosis

Anxiety

The long-term effects of magic mushroom use will require more research. However, some studies have shown that long-term changes in character and flashbacks are common. Their use can cause more harm that good as magic mushrooms are similar to noxious mushrooms. It can cause serious illnesses, organ diseases, death, and even death. It is essential for magic mushroom items not to be tainted. Pharm Chem Street Drug Laboratory investigated 886 samples claimed to have been psilocybin. Of these, only 252 (28%) showed signs of psychoactive effects. Meanwhile, 275 (31%), were regular mushrooms that had been grown locally and bound with LSD/phencyclidine (PCP), while 328 (37%) contained no medication.

Help with Mushroom Poisoning

If you are concerned that your loved one has eaten a poisonous or poisonous mushroom, contact the poison control department in your area.

Use indications

These are signs that you may be exposed to magic mushrooms. Consider any movement in rest and eating due to medication. Also, consider movements in character, temperament, and social skills.

Common Questions & Myths

There are many myths around magic mushrooms. They are said to be "more secure" than other hallucinogenics, and offer a milder experience. Magic mushrooms have the potential to inflict more harm than others and are as unpredictable as other drugs in their "class". A few people have reported having more serious and disturbing mental issues from magic mushrooms than LSD. Various individuals have tested and compared the chemical compound in fly agaric mushrooms with psilocybin-containing mushrooms; they are not equivalent. Fly agaric fungi contain psychoactive synthetic substances that have been known to cause jerking.

* Resilience.

Magic mushrooms have the same effect as other drugs. They are more resilient than normal drugs and can be difficult to resist. This means that you will need to consume more mushrooms to have the same impact. It is possible to develop resilience with mushrooms. This can happen because you can burn through large amounts of the substance, which can lead to glut manifestations. This can include tumult or spewing, muscle shortcoming and frenzy or neurosis.

Psilocybin won't make you a habit and will not lead to a pattern of use. The medication can cause a remarkable "trip." Individuals may be able to build resilience to the medication fairly quickly. However, it will not take long before they start to feel any effect.

Withdrawal

Psilocybin users rarely report withdrawal symptoms. Some users experience mental issues that may lead to depression.

How long can Psilocybin remain in your system for?

Although the transient effects of magic mushrooms typically subside within 6 to 12 hours however, users can experience long-term changes in their personality and flashbacks. The typical psilocybin middle-experience takes between one and two hours. However, it can take up to six hours for the drug to be completely out of your system. The majority of pee drug testing methods don't detect psilocybin within a person's body. However, you can request specific tests to check for this amazing stimulant. Magic mushrooms are similar to hard drugs and can be found within hair follicles up to 90 days.

How to Get Assistance

It is a good idea to have a discussion about the dangers of hallucinogenic drugs with anyone you know who uses magic mushrooms. It is important to let them know you are there for support. To help you and your loved ones who are struggling with addiction or substance use, please contact the Substance Abuse and Mental Health Services Administration.

Chapter 8: Using Agar

In general, your mushroom culture should be grown on agar plates with nutrients. Agar is known for its ability to produce radial and two-dimensional growth patterns. This allows for easy analysis of your culture to determine if any contamination has occurred. Agar's molecular structure is similar to that of sugar. You can see the similarities when it's dissolved in water. Then, let it cool in water. The agar isn't nutritious for the yeast so it must be infused with yeast extract. Combine the ingredients in a container with heat resistance. Heat sterilize the mixture using a pressure cook and then strain them into Petri dishes. MYA (Malt-Yeast Extract Agar) is the most widely used agar media to help fungus.

Senescence

The culture can age and degrade over time. You will notice that strains can senescence. Sometimes, culture may not grow or show signs of growth after repeated transfers from one plate onto another. This could be bad or good. It's unclear what causes this. However, it occurs when cultures are kept in the exact same substrate recipe for too much time. Your fungi, in other words, would like to have variety when it came to food. This is why it is important to make sure your recipe has variations. This will ensure that the fungus is constantly challenged and creates new enzymes in response. You can do this by adding some grain flour in each batch of flour, and changing the types you use to make new plates.

It is also a good idea for your shrooms to be grown with entirely new media. This is ideal if you have an old culture that's dying out and you want to bring back its life. Get rid of any starch and simple carbohydrates once this happens. It will take some time before it can grow in this new medium. However, within a few weeks, it will begin to grow again on MYA. It can be fed peanut butter or jam, soybeans, and even paper pellets. If your plant isn't growing on one of these, try switching to another. Be careful how often you transfer your culture because it can cause destruction. Instead of creating a whole new generation, you can just make multiple copies of the old cultures and store them indefinitely until you are ready.

Making Malt Yeast Agar

You'll Need:

* 1 gram yeast Extract

* 12g of light malt extract

* 22g agar

* 1 Liter of tapwater

* 1.4 teaspoon organic wheat flour. You can also add rice, rye and amaranth to this recipe.

* 5g wood fuel pellets

* 8mL of 3% hydrogen peroxide (optional and not necessary after the sterilization and cooling procedures as detailed in the instructions below).

Steps:

1. All dry ingredients should be taken out and placed in a glass jar. Add in the water.

Be sure to use only one-half or more of the media. It will boil if you sterilize it. You should ensure that the neck of the bottle has been closed. You can use cotton yarn to do this. Next, wrap your neck with aluminum foil.

2. Place the jar and sufficient water in your pressure cooker. When working with hydrogen Peroxide, make sure to sterilize at least 2 pipettes. Wrap them in aluminum so they are sterile until you use them.

3. Sterilize it for 30 minutes at 15 Psi. You should make sure that you don't let the agar cook for more than 45 mins. That will cause it to caramelize. To be safe, use a potholder as you transport things from your pressure kettle to your work area.

4. Peroxide: Once your jar has cooled enough on the outside to allow you to handle it, and the temperature is between 120 and 140 degrees Fahrenheit inside, add 8 mL. Use a measuring spoon or pipette. Use a whisk to mix the medium.

Don't overdo the mixing as you don't want bubbles to form.

5. Petri dishes can be opened up and stacked on the right side. Keep the plastic wrap for later, so you can store them once you're done.

6. Do ten dishes at one time. The entire stack can be lifted using the bottom plate. This will allow the top half to remain on the bench. Slowly pour the medium that you require onto the plate. Allow it to completely cover the stack. Then, place the stack on top of the medium and repeat until you're finished. It should take approximately 20-30 100 mm Petri dish dishes to be filled with your medium. Use gentleness when you pour the mixture. Pay attention to any solids at bottom to make sure you don't accidentally pour them in.

7. If the agar begins to harden, do not use it.

8. Once the plates are finished, arrange them in an orderly fashion and then remove the sleeves. This will allow the

plates to cool down slowly and evenly. This avoids the possibility of condensation. Condensation can make it hard to see the gel and could lead to contamination. A sterilized mug, or a heavy glass filled full of hot water can be used to cover each stack.

9. Let all plates cool down overnight.

10. Plates that contain peroxide are good for a few more days. As long as there are no drafts and they are kept somewhere cool so you can get rid any condensation. They should be placed in stacks of approximately three each and covered with wax paper. If they have no peroxide, make sure to put them right in their sleeves as soon a possible.

11. Your plastic sleeve should be slipped back onto the plates. Then, use clear tape for sealing them. Place them on their sides to prevent condensation. Keep them dry.

The anything Agar Medium is the medium for reviving your cultural heritage. Here's the way to do it.

You'll Need:

* 1 liter of water from the tap

* 22g of agar

* 20g of...anything (use any of the suggestions).

* 8 mL Hydrogen peroxide (3 percent) (you need to add this in after you have sterilized).

Steps:

1. Make a powder from the ground material. A blender can be used to puree the mixture in water.

2. Follow the same steps that were followed for making your MYA.

Caring for Your Cultures, Dishes

To prevent contaminants from getting to your cultures when you transfer them, make sure the lids are only removed for a few seconds and keep them above the plate. Place your cultures on top of the agar. Give the transfers time to completely grow onto the new plates before flipping them upside down. Also, wrap the culture plates in parafilm.

Spore Streaking

When you are not using the PF Tek for your cubensis growth, you can start the cultures by working with spores. You could use the traditional method. Use a sterilized inoculation loop and pick a few spores off your print. Run them through a streak on your plate of Agar. Petri dishes with peroxide can be used, but you should not use them. This would kill your spores. Rush Wayne's method also works, which is a good thing. Because the discs have small openings and the test tubes have narrow openings you won't have to worry about contaminants. This is especially true if you don't use peroxide. This is a faster way to colonize the print. Additionally, the disc acts as both the substrate for the spores and the tool for removing them from it. It is also very efficient for transferring them if the print doesn't have enough.

You can cut out small discs by using a hole puncher from a flat piece or cardboard. Then, moisten the discs a little and then put them in your jar. You should sterilize your spores and test tubes with five to 10 drops of your MYA liquid. Once everything has cooled down, you can pull out your spores using the discs. You'll see your spores develop over time. When they've colonized discs, you should transfer them onto agar plates with peroxide.

The Agar Spore Method

You'll do the exact same thing as you did with your sporewater syringes but this time, your spores are transferred to agar plates.

You'll Need:

* Parafilm

* Alcohol lamp

* Spore print

* Inoculating syringe

* Agar Petri dishes (peroxide free)

Steps:

1. Use your glove or flow hood to warm up the inoculation valve inside your alcohol-lamp. Let it heat to a high temperature.

2. With your free hand raise your petri plate and push your loop's tip in the middle of the Agaric to allow it to cool down. This will allow a thin agar coating to form on the loop. It is this that the spores latch onto.

3. Cover the plate. Cover the plate with the loop and grab some spores. The amount you need is very minimal.

4. The spores can be moved from the print onto your petri dishes by streaking them, almost as if you were writing the letter S.

5. Your loop should be sterilized once more. Wait for the loop to cool before you start streaking next plates. Always sterilize from one plate to the next.

6. Use parafilm to cover your plates once you're done with inoculating. Your marker can be used to add the required data to your plates. Then let incubation take place with the agar on top.

Sporegermination with Cardboard Discs
You'll Need:
* Spore print
* Parafilm
* Tweezers
* Jar with lid (half a pint).
* Eyedropper (or pipette)
* Test tubes or Vials with Screw Caps (Use 2 to 4 for each Spore Print)
* Cardboard disks

* Alcohol lamp

* MYA solution (100mL Water, a very small pinch yeast extract, and 1 tablespoon of malt)

Steps:

1. Half-pint jar: Pour 1 to 2 ML water into the jar. Cover the jar with your cardboard pieces and seal it.

2. Now it's time for sterilization of your tubes and containers. For about 15 minutes, repeat this process. At 45 psi, maintain this pressure. Let it cool completely.

3. Place all of the material you plan to use in your gloves box.

4. You can light an alcohol lamp and heat a pair or tweezers. Then let them cool.

5. Open your jar. Take out a disc with tweezers. Cover it again.

6. Touch the disc until you see your sporeprint. You don't need to touch anything but the edge. To ensure the spores stick, you need to lean in close.

7. You can open a tube to place the disc.

8. Do this three to a maximum of five times for each tube. Also, make sure that you make at most two tubes for each of the spore prints.

9. Seal your tubes using parafilm Let them incubate.

10. After the colonization process has ended, transfer them onto peroxided agar plates.

The Incubation Process

Incubation should be done somewhere that is warm and free from wind currents. Keep the temperature at between 75 and 86 degrees Fahrenheit. If you are storing them in the room's normal temperature, you can put them in a plastic container or box. Otherwise, you need an incubator.

Cloning

For a new culture, you can use freshly harvested mushrooms. You will end up with a single strain which looks very similar to the parent, which is what makes it called a clone. It's important to choose the best specimens because they will give the best clones. Once you have found the right one, you simply need to cut or tear the shrooms out of your glove box. Then take some of the mycelium off and place it onto a new agarplate. After a while the mycelium can begin to grow.

Sometimes, clones of parents will look very different in mycelial than the parent. This is why it is important to keep several cultures. Although it can be easy to assume it's doing well, not all varieties will. The chances are that the cells inside the shrooms will be sterile as they haven't been exposed the elements or environment. To make sure they stay sterile, please do the cloning right after you pick them up. If that's not possible, they should be kept in a cold, dry place, and stored in Tupperware. Tupperware must be wrapped in a piece of paper towel. It is best to keep them in your refrigerator for no longer than two days.

Peroxide has many benefits when it comes to cloning. Peroxide should be used to treat the agar you are using for tissue culture.

You'll Need:

* Alcohol lamp

* Alcohol

* Mushrooms

* Peroxide Petri dishes

* Paper towels (or cotton balls).

* Scalpel

Steps:

1. Your mushrooms should be cleaned. Get rid of any loose material from the casing. Please do it somewhere other than your workspace.

2. Take a cotton ball and soak it in alcohol. Then, use the cotton ball to clean the shrooms. You can do this in the glove box.

3. You can sterilize your scalpel by lighting the lamp. Gently squeeze the stipe with your thumb and forefinger. Cut along the length and cut down the middle. Now you can open up the mushroom to reveal two halves. Cut the cap. Don't touch the surface from which you are making a clone. It could infect the tissue.

4. You should sterilize your knife every time it is used.

5. Use your Petri dish to add some mycelium from the shroom's cap. The material should be as large as possible, approximately three to eight mm in length and width. As it may be contaminated, please don't cut your shroom beyond the exposed portion.

6. Use the tip of your scalpel to slice the mycelium gently. Place the petri dish's lid on your other side. Next, place the cut piece in the middle. If the mycelium sticks onto your scalpel you can attempt to cut it while pushing into the Agagar.

7. Continue the process with all three plates.

8. You can seal the plates using parafilm. Once that's done, you can put them in an incubator. They should be flipped over once they start growing.

It will take days or up to one week for growth to happen. Subculture it as soon and as possible.

Subculture Process
You'll Need:
* Parafilm, alcohol lamp

* Agar cultures
* Scalpel
* Sterile agar plates

Steps:

1. You can find the parafilm in your glovebox.

2. You can heat the scalpel's edge with an alcohol lamp. Wait until it turns red. Let it cool in an oven-safe dish.

3. Take the lid from the prime culture and use it to make squares or wedges. This should yield approximately 1 centimeter of material. You can reduce the desired number of wedges.

4. Remove the lid completely from the culture plate. Then, with your knife, lift the plate's lid slightly to one end. Begin by piercing one of your agar slivers or wedges with the tip end of your knife. Then, place the new dish in its middle, making sure that it is face-down.

5. For each dish, do the same, seal them, and then use a marker to make notes about it. It is best to store it upside down.

Contamination

You can't avoid contamination. This is why two-dimensional plates with agar are so useful. Sometimes it may be necessary to save contaminated materials if you're not careful about replicating transfers or staying clean. If this is the case you should take the contaminated part out of the plate and move it into a different one. Don't try and remove all the contaminants from the plates, as they could become contaminated once more. You might have to do this multiple times before you can completely remove the mold. Here's how we can find out what caused the contamination.

1. The possibility of contamination before you use the dishes could indicate that the agar wasn't sterilized adequately or that the contamination occurred while you were storing the agar or pouring it onto the plates. There could be a problem with the peroxide level in your agar.

2. If the contamination is visible around the edges of the dish, such as a full-ring or unique colonies appearing, it could be

because the unsterilized air was cooling. Be sure to let the agar cool completely before pouring. Once the dish is cool, you can cover it with your sleeves.

3. If the contamination occurs at the point where the inoculation was performed, it indicates that the parent-culture was contaminated. It may also be possible that the inoculation tool or knife used was not completely sterilized. Be sure to heat them until the red color is achieved.

4. If you see something shiny and clear that is bright yellow, pink, or green, it's likely you have bacteria. They are drawn to dampness so condensation might be on the dish's covers. Make sure the agar is cool before pouring. Let the dishes cool inside their sleeves. Be sure to cover the dish with the agar.

Storing Strains on the Long Haul

Once you have a healthy variety, it's a good idea for you to continue to propagate it. Do your best to avoid senescence. Only transfer the cultures that have been used a lot. You should keep one main culture of every strain. This is what you keep in your refrigerator for long-term use to make subcultures, if necessary.

Keep your culture at about 38 degrees Fahrenheit. It is possible to bring them back alive by placing them on a new plate. This will allow them to develop into a subculture. Place your cultures in sterilized glass tubes with sterilized pellets of paper. If they are kept on agar, there is a risk that they will die from too much sugar. You can also use a half-pint glass jar to test them. When they are ready to be transferred, they can be placed in a plastic baggie.

Storing with Paper Pellets

You'll Need:

* Tap water
* A funnel
* Paper pellet cat litter
* Test tubes

Steps:

1. Take your paper pellets out of the bag and moisten them. You want them to reach field capacity.

2. Fill the tubes approximately a third to halfway. It is important to get rid of any agar on the outside. These should be covered with loose sheets.

3. You can sterilize the containers by heating them at 15 PSI for 30 minutes in a pressure cooker. You can stack the bottles in layers but you should place your tubes on a stand to ensure they are upright. If you don't possess a rack you can simply place the tubes inside a metal can.

4. Allow the cooker time to cool. It should be warm to touch. Transfer the containers to a glove box and let them cool.

How to Innoculate Your Tubs

1. You can disinfect the scalpel with a flame. Repeat this process for the tube's neck.

2. A little bit of the healthy culture's agar can be taken out. Keep your sawdust tube horizontally. Put the agar shard on the tube's upper side and gently tap it into sawdust.

3. Cover the container, cover the cap or lid with parafilm, mark as required. Allow this

to incubate for a few hours. Then transfer the tubes into another container (like a Ziploc, Tupperware, or Ziploc) and put them in a refrigerator.

4. It is easy to recover your culture. All you have to do it let the culture rest at room temperature 2 days. After that, use a sterilized environment to transfer a small piece mycelium colonized paper to a fresh, peroxide-treated agar plate.

Chapter 9: Grains, Fruiting Pots And Casing Sol

Preparing Your Grain Spawn

Grain spawn is a whole-grain cooked with some calcium sulfurate and calcium carbonate. The former buffers the pH of the grains, while the latter keeps them separate. The fungus absorbs both minerals and pH buffers. It is best to cook the rice and then soak it overnight in hot, salted water. Any whole grain, including wheat, rye, corn, and rye with large kernels is possible to use. Winter wheat is recommended because it's low in bacterial endospores. Additionally, it cooks evenly.

Steps:

1. You should use a pot that is big enough. The grain will expand when it is cooked. To ensure that it doesn't double in size, make sure to use a pot with a capacity of three and add water. The water should contain twice as much grain. Let it boil before

adding the dry grains. After that, boil it until it becomes liquid.

2. Allow it to heat for ten seconds, then turn off. Let it sit in the pot for eight hours and then let it cool. The grain should be at least twice its original volume. You can crush the grain with your fingers to determine if it's set. It should feel soft throughout.

3. Drain the grain with a colander. Are they sticky or wet? Wash them with cold water. Then drain them.

4. Put the grain and the calcium carbonate and calcium sulfate into the containers. You can seal the containers and give them a good shake before putting them in the pressure cooker. You need to leave space around each container. Also, you will need a pipette so you can measure your peroxide.

5. Sterilize 15 minutes

6. Let it cool completely. It might be necessary to let it rest overnight. The inoculated cells should be kept in the sealed oven until they are ready for use.

Transferring from Agar - Grain

Inoculating small portions of the grain can be done with agar cultures. For 6 quart-sized jars, you can use one plate as a colonizer. To protect against contaminants, the grain will have peroxide added when it is inoculated. You should add 6mL of water to each cup.

You'll Need:

* 10ml measuring scoop or pipette
* Agar culture
* Alcohol lamp
* 3 percent hydrogen peroxide
* Grain jars (sterilized)
* Scalpel

Steps:

1. Take the jars and put them in your glovebox.

2. Take off the caps of the jars but keep them on the container. Measure the hydrogen peroxide required and add it to each jar. Be sure to keep the lid on top. Secure them.

3. Give each container a thorough shake. This will separate grains and ensure the

peroxide reaches every part of the jar. Take off the lid and keep it in place. After the lid has been removed, you can put the jar down gently, ensuring that the grain is not disturbed. Do the same with the rest of your jars.

4. Let the knife cool in a glass of water before sterilizing it.

5. Make sure to cut your culture dish into pieces or wedges. Each jar should have at most two. Please be careful not to cut into the parent mycelium at the top of the plate.

6. Your scalpel's tip should be used to make a wedge. Cover the plate with the cover and let the wedge fall onto your grain. With the mycelium facing down, place the wedge in direct contact with your grain. To loosen the square, press gently on the jar's outside rim.

7. Do the same with another square. Once you have done that, place the cover back on your jar.

8. After inoculating every jar, screw them tightly shut and gently tap on them to

force the grains to cover all of the agar pieces. Please do not shake the jars.

9. Mark the containers with your marker. Place them in the incubation zone.

Inoculating with Syringes

For this, you do not need hydrogen peroxide.

1. After sterilizing the grain, let it cool in the jars. Then, take them to the glove box.

2. Do not pull the covers off of the jars.

3. After removing the cover, clean the needle with a cotton soaked in alcohol. Once the needle is red, light the alcohol lamp to make it glow. Let it cool off for a few more seconds.

4. To inject your spore solutions into the grain, open each container one at a.

5. Cover the container, shake it, and allow it to incubate.

How to Incubate Your Jars

Your incubator might not be large enough for all of your jars. If you don't want to spend the money on new ones, or if they are too expensive, you can keep them safe and warm. A closet shelf is a good place.

Keep the temperature between 65 and 82 degrees Fahrenheit. Your mycelium will grow normally, but a bit slower. When mycelium eats the substrate, it generates heat. It's often enough to raise the temperature a little. To avoid overheating, it's better not to work at the upper end of this temperature range.

Boosting Growth

Every now and again, shake the grain cultures to increase their speed and uniformity. After one week or less, the mycelium has moved from the agar pieces to the grain to colonize. Once they are about an inch in diameter, you can shake it. Be gentle when shaking it. The aim is to get the grains apart and make sure they are even. You want to make sure that the grains are evenly broken up. The more colonization happens, the more individual grains will stick together. Instead, you can use a thick towel to support the pillow.

Ideally, two shakes should be given to the jars when the colonization has completed. This can be done one week. After the first attempt, the mycelium will become invisible and it will seem like nothing is taking place. But give it a couple days and they'll colonize at more locations than before.

Grain Contamination

Always be on the lookout for contamination. Take a look at what happens to the jars after you shake them. Although some jars look clean, you may discover contamination after a few days. If your mycelium fails to colonize again within 24 hours or the process is slow, then bacteria has infiltrated. They might appear as small spots or wet bubbles surrounding the grains. You might also see them in the inner part. It might smell like rotten or sour apples. This is an indication of fermentation. You will easily be able see if it's mold.

It is important to remove the bad ones as soon you detect contamination in your grain-spawn. If you don't do this, you will have billions more mold spores. You can pressure cook the contaminated bottles before you open them. This will ensure that no contaminants make it into the sterilized environment of your laboratory. If you do not want to do that please put the contents of the container somewhere other than your lab. After you have returned to your space, wash your clothing and take a bath.

Transferring Grain to Grain

Use fully colonized grain container immediately after you get them. If they aren't used within 14 days or a week, your chances of success will decrease. You can inoculate new vessels with smaller containers of grain. A container of grain could be enough to produce ten new containers or four larger ones. Although you can make more spawn with the new generations, it is better to keep them to three generations or less.

You can use the grain bowls to inoculate either the fruiting-agar or the fruit yourself. If you need more spawn to work with, you only need to transfer one grain to another. Select the best specimens possible for your transfer. Because they are healthier than the others, it is easy to identify which ones you should use. If anyone appears weak or slow to grow, you should not use any of the uncolonized grains or wet spots. Make sure you shake them well again before letting them incubate. If the cultures are healthy, they should return stronger with mycelia. Note that grain to grain transfer is done the same way as an "agar transfer". Once you have sterilized the grain containers, you add some of your colonized grain. How many containers you have to inoculate will dictate how much spawn to add. Split them evenly. You can seal, shake and incubate your new jars.

Containers for large spawn

For spawns larger than a half a gallon, you can use autoclavablespawn bags. With a standard size of 18 inches by 8 inches by 4 inches, you will be able get ten-fold the grain from a quart container. Additionally, the bag won't take up as much space in your incubator or pressure cooker. Because the bag can be flexible, you can easily examine the seed and manipulate it as many times you need. It's also much easier for you to tear the grain apart.

Bags are inoculated using jars and other large containers. It is best to inoculate the bags from jars or other large containers. A large amount of inoculating matter should be used for each bag to speed up the process. The amount of inoculating material needed for each bag should be about 1 cup of already colonized rice. A quart jar filled with inoculated material is sufficient for two to four bags.

Bags have the disadvantage of being difficult to keep sterile. Also, it's more difficult to inoculate multiple people at once. You'll need to inoculate your flowhood, which should be large and HEPA. You may want to check that all bags contain peroxide if you don't already have it. To seal the bags across top, use an impulse sealer. Make a few passes that are separated by a few mm.

Make sure you don't get too much moisture into your large containers. The mycelium can absorb all of it, so the smaller containers can be fine with less water. This could pose a problem when using large quantities of grain because the mycelium could become suffocated. This is why it's better to use more calcium and gypsum.

This will prevent the grain from becoming too wet. This can easily be avoided by soaking your grain in hot, not boiling water. Make sure to drain the grain well before you use. Additionally, if your container is too wet while you are making it, you may add more gypsum. Gypsum will absorb all the moisture. You want the grain dried when you touch the grain.

Grain Bags - Loading and Cooking

1. You can fill your bags with air and press the empty spaces to get rid of all the air. The flab should be folded under the bag.

2. Place the bags in your pressure cooker. To do this, keep the filter pieces out of the way and make sure that there's enough

space between each bag. To raise the bags off the bottom of your cooker, you can use a trivet. Make sure that they don't touch the sides or the sides of any pot. Use peroxide to sterilize the pot. To do this, put a graduated tube in the pan.

How to Innoculate Your Grain Bags

1. Let everything cool down before you take it to the work place.

2. Make sure to shake the culture jar before you attempt to break up the colony.

3.   Measure   80mL   with   a pipette/graduated cylinder

4. You need to quickly open the bag. Pour the peroxide inside and then fold the flap down so the air doesn't get in. Make sure to fold it several more times.

5. You can give the bag a gentle shake by holding it in your hands. Keep it shut in your work area.

6. Do the exact same thing for all the bags.

7. Open one bag, add your colonized grain, fold the flap, and then do the same with all of the remaining bags.

179

8. Grab your impulse-sealer and seal the bags. Give it a couple more swipes.

9. Give the bag some time to shake it. After that, you can use your market and take notes of any important information.

Fruiting Containers

Next, once your substrate is fully colonized you will need to find a container suitable for fruiting or casing. It all comes down to how many fruits you wish to grow. If you're working with smaller amounts or grain, the substrate should be at least 2 to 3 in depth. For larger amounts, 6 inches is the recommended depth. Make sure you choose one made from a material strong enough that it can hold the substrate in its place while colonization takes place. It should also have an opaque layer so that light falls only on the soil. It is important that the container's height should not exceed the depth of the substrate.

Some growers choose containers that have covers that can be snipped on to induce humidity. However you must drill holes in the container's sides to allow for airflow. Instead, consider using opaque or shallow containers that have enough light. Your fruiting room doesn't have to look so extravagant. This could be a clear, plastic bag that has holes cut in it to allow for airflow. This bag can be placed in front of a window with sufficient sunlight. For more storage, you can buy a shelf with multiple levels to accommodate all your containers. You will need fluorescent lights and a humidifier to make the shelf work.

You can also use the plastic dishwashing tubs. The dimensions of this tub are 11.5"x13.5"x7". This will hold between 4 and 8 quart-sized bottles or a bag full of grain. You will need to work more substrate if the containers are larger than 20 inches by 15 inches by 7 inches deep.

Humidity Tent

These containers need to be kept moist in order to prevent moisture from getting into the substrate and casing. Cubensis can tolerate low humidity levels up to 70 percent. Keep the container placed in a small place and water well.

You can also put smaller trays inside the bags, tie them up and punch holes in the sides and top to allow for airflow. The holes should not exceed four to five per square foot and each one no more than half an in. You can also buy pre-perforated bags. It's important to make sure that the container is removed from the bag before you mist to help displace any CO_2 gasses. The bags must have sufficient space to allow the mushrooms grow. It should take approximately 9 inches.

You can store the container in a clear storage tub made of plastic. Invert it with holes on the sides for airflow. Alternately, you can use a "tented shelf", which is a shelf that has been wrapped in plastic with a zip for humidity. These can be purchased from garden supply stores. These shelves are big enough for small containers and whole tubs.

Maintain Humidity levels

You should keep the smaller fruiting container in plastic bags with holes. The larger ones should be stored inside large clear bags. You can also keep them in multiples on a growing rack. You will need to ensure the humidity is equal to the substrate the mushrooms are held in. Also, it should be easy for you to keep the moisture at the correct levels by misting your shrooms every day. Your casing should be moist enough to evaporate into your air and enable the mushrooms to grow. If your air is too dry you'll need a humidifier. This is available at your local department stores. This can be done by placing the dehumidifier in one of your shelves. It is possible for condensation to form so it is important that you have a large tray in the bottom of your rack. To prevent mold growth, please empty the tray and sterilize it often.

Let's discuss lighting

A lighting arrangement that matches your fruiting space is essential. Psilocybes mushrooms are different than plants because they only require light to promote growth, and not to obtain nutrition or energy. They also only need light for fruiting. This works best if you have enough light to see clearly in your grow space. It might not be enough to light one tub or several PF jars. For large grow racks you will need compact fluorescent lights of around 15 to 20% watts. Be sure to keep them out of the grow chamber. They can affect temperature and may cause a short circuit. Depending upon the size and number of containers you have, you might need to place multiple lamps at different points so that your culture doesn't get shadowed. You only need to set your lights on timers as your shrooms require about 8 hours of daylight each day.

www.ingramcontent.com/pod-product-compliance
Lightning Source LLC
Chambersburg PA
CBHW060222030426
42335CB00014B/1315